HEALTHY YOU, HEALTHY TEAM, HEALTHY COMPANY

HEALTHY YOU

HEALTHY TEAM

HEALTHY COMPANY

HOW TO IMPLEMENT AN EMPLOYEE WELLNESS PROGRAM INTO YOUR ORGANIZATION

JOSHUA DETILLIO

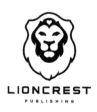

LIONCREST
PUBLISHING

HEALTHY YOU, HEALTHY TEAM, HEALTHY COMPANY
How to Implement an Employee Wellness Program in Your Organization

ISBN   978-1-5445-1083-5 *Paperback*
        978-1-5445-1082-8 *Ebook*

I dedicate this book to my loving wife, Consuelo, my better half, who started me on my journey toward healthy living many years ago.

CONTENTS

ACKNOWLEDGMENTS

Writing a book about this journey toward healthy living has been a team effort. I am very fortunate to be surrounded by some truly amazing people who have helped, supported, and educated me along the way.

Thank you to my team at Gulf Coast Medical Center. I have seen leaders, physicians, and employees begin journeys toward healthy living and self-care. Thank you for letting me test various initiatives and strategies, and always know I did it all because I truly care about you and your health.

Finally, I'd like to dedicate this book to my incredible family. Thank you to my mom, dad, brother, sister, and extended family for the love and support you have always given me. All of you have been role models and have taught me so much. Most importantly, I'd like to thank my wife, Consuelo. You have given your whole life to supporting me and our family. Without your love and support, I would not be able to pursue my dreams or be able to write a book. I am so lucky to have you as a soul mate, and I love you with all of my heart. To my wonderful children, Valentina and Luca, you inspire me to be the best me. Always remember, your Daddy loves you.

PROLOGUE

MY STORY

I was born in 1975, part of Generation X. We were the first generation that had access to fast food, and we grew up on much more processed food than any previous generation. When we were kids, we would go to McDonald's once a week if we were good; a Happy Meal was our "reward."

Growing up in this context, I never truly took time to think about food. I heard everyone say to eat your fruits and vegetables, but I assumed exercise would cancel out any negative effects of a poor diet. I started swimming very young—around age five—and swam all the way through college. Because I was working out and swimming all of the time, I never had a problem with my weight. I could eat large helpings of pizza, pasta, and fast food, and never gain a pound. As an athlete, I was encouraged to eat a lot.

The first time I took notice of what I was eating was when I went to the US Military Academy at West Point. I continued to swim and continued to eat a lot, but when the off-season came around, I began to gain weight for the first time. When you are eighteen or nineteen, you can keep weight off by working out, so lifting weights in the gym worked as a simple fix when I needed it. The real problem, however, was that I still was not eating well.

It took words from a friend I respected to finally shake me out of my ignorance. Derek was a year ahead of me, and I viewed him as a mentor. He was a swimmer, and we worked out together all the time. I'll always remember one night when we were eating together, and he passed me the broccoli. When I said I didn't want any, he furrowed his brow, and I could see in his eyes that he was not happy with me. For the first time ever, I truly considered the amount of vegetables I was or wasn't eating.

His response got me thinking about my eating habits in general. Of course, my parents had always told me to eat my vegetables as well, but we don't always listen to our parents. When Derek said, "You need to eat your vegetables. What are you thinking?" I took his words to heart. I needed that little boost from an authority figure in my life, at a critical age, when I was forming many of my lifelong habits.

In the Army, we focused on getting enough calories for ourselves and our soldiers to have plenty of energy for the mission or whatever training we were doing. We didn't always follow the best diet, but my time in the Army helped me realize that food is a tool for energy. You may have heard the well-known phrase: "Some people live to eat, and some people eat to live." During these years, I woke up to the fact that I could eat to live by eating more simply. That one reality influenced many of my choices later in life.

When I got out of the Army, I started working in hospitals. I ate what I felt was a fairly healthy diet: limiting sugar, soft drinks, and overall calories. I thought I was doing well until I went to Harvard to get my master's degree in public health. Back in 2007, there was very little being written about nutrition. The movement around healthy eating was not yet in full effect, and I discovered there was so much more to learn. I finished the master's program wanting to know more, but not knowing where to look to find answers.

This feeling was compounded when I went back to work at a hospital in West Palm Beach and started seeing a lot of younger adults experiencing serious chronic illnesses like strokes, heart attacks, and even cancer. Many of them were in their thirties—close to my age. I started wondering: *What is going on? Why are these young adults getting chronic diseases?* I was able to file the questions away in the back of my mind for a short time, until both of my parents were diagnosed with chronic diseases. That's when I couldn't simply move past the thought that something was not right.

At the same time my parents were experiencing major health concerns, I was transitioning into a new job as chief administrative officer of Gulf Coast Medical Center in Fort Myers. With everything that was happening, I became incredibly stressed. When I started gaining weight, I tried to go back to my normal fix of working out more. This time around, though, I couldn't lose all the weight through exercise alone. I was significantly heavier than I had ever been, and I needed to do something differently.

My motivation was not only to lose weight; I wanted to improve my athletic and workout performance as well. I began hearing about athletes modifying their diets and eating more simply. Since I continued to be an athlete—swimming and running, doing CrossFit, and participating in triathlons—these stories really piqued my interest.

The first book I picked up was *Thrive* by Brendan Brazier. It's a phenomenal book that I always recommend to others because of how much it impacted me. Brendan focuses on a plant-based, whole-foods diet that helps you achieve optimal performance in both athletics and life. So that was where I started. I went cold turkey from day one. I told myself I was going to do exactly what the book said, and I did it.

It helped to have a colleague at work, Scott, who was also an athlete and was committed to getting healthy and staying young with me. We would compete in triathlons together and often bounce ideas off of each other about food and wellness. Since we were both in leadership positions, we began to discuss how we could promote wellness within our organization.

ON THE FRONTLINES OF HEALTHCARE

All of us who work in healthcare got into the industry so that we could help people. Still, it's strange how healthy eating is an afterthought in hospitals—a topic that is rarely addressed. I have witnessed firsthand as patients recovering from a heart attack come out of surgery and have bacon and eggs for breakfast the next morning. It's as if there is no consideration about what food is doing to our bodies in the very place that focuses on the healing of bodies.

Another interesting phenomenon in the healthcare

world is that the workforce doesn't always practice what it preaches. Doctors, nurses, and hospital staff care about health and wellness from a philosophical standpoint, but food and wellness choices are rarely discussed. These are viewed as personal topics, like politics or religion.

While you might think our organization, a hospital, would be more open to an employee wellness program, we have experienced many of the same obstacles as any other organization. I had to learn to tread lightly—to set the example by living a healthy life. In this way, I could help others when they were ready to make changes.

THE GREATER MISSION

Throughout this journey of developing an employee wellness program, we have helped a lot of people—certainly employees, but also patients and others in our community. We also realized that there are many more people out there whom we could be helping. That was the impetus behind this book and its message. It's exciting to know that we live in a perfect time for this message to be received.

A significant movement is building around wellness, food, and prevention. People are starting to get curious. The baby boomers who are entering their seventies are developing multiple chronic illnesses, taking ten to fifteen medications, and generally not thriving in their golden years. As a society, we are starting to question what is going on. Millennials, in particular, are questioning everything. Your employees are ready for answers.

Working in a hospital, I see disease every day. I have seen forty-year-old fathers come in—with wives and kids at home—and not make it after a heart attack. It didn't take long for me to start asking, "What if?" What if that guy could have been saved? Would he be safe at home with his family if he had better understood food and wellness earlier in his life? Our mission has come from these kinds of questions. It is simple: we want to save more lives.

Despite our country's abundance of unhealthy food and an increase in chronic diseases, I hope to build awareness that you don't have to continue to suffer. You and your family can be healthier and stay out of the hospital altogether. And yes, in spite of working in a hospital, I'd rather you stay out of one.

In this book, we will explore how an employee wellness program can offer many benefits for you and your company. In the end, though, it all boils down to the greater mission: More people can be helped. More lives can be saved.

INTRODUCTION

WELLNESS IS A WIN-WIN

I am on a mission to be healthy and help others be healthy. It is a mission that is close to my heart and likely close to yours if you are reading this book. However, this mission, no matter how noble it may be, is often limited in its impact until it turns into a movement that is sustained by numbers.

If you are a leader in your company, you have an opportunity to create a movement toward greater health in the world by developing an employee wellness program. This program will empower a large group of people to live healthier lives, at the same time benefiting your company as well.

Many companies have good intentions when it comes to

wellness programs. Some have even seen a level of success with their programs, but few have looked at metrics or trends in their employee populations. Companies like Google, IBM, and American Express have gone to great lengths to make gyms, healthier foods, standing desks, on-site doctors and medical care, and meditation areas available to their employees. While those large companies led the way, I wanted to do all those things and more. As soon as I started working at our hospital, I had the feeling that we could be doing more to encourage wellness.

Perhaps you are also hoping to revamp what has been done in your organization up to this point, or you might be considering launching a brand-new program. No matter your status, this book will give you a roadmap for success. You will gain the knowledge you need to provide your employees with the right resources, opportunities, and motivation to improve their health.

As you begin, remember that some of these changes will take time, especially if you are developing a program in a large organization. When I started at our hospital, we had around two thousand employees altogether, and that number has risen over the past few years. Because we were hoping to make a real impact, we focused on incremental changes that would steer a big ship, little by little, over time. We chose to focus on the food that is offered in our hospitals. At times, progress has seemed slow, but focusing on this single objective has yielded incredible results.

After years of developing our program, we now have a captive audience among employees, but that wasn't always the case. We had to gain their trust and learn what would truly inspire them to improve their health. Now, even our patients (the customers of our business) are directly affected by our employees' stories.

You might be wondering: *Isn't a hospital the place people come to get better? Wouldn't healthy living be a focus by default?* Strangely enough, food is often an afterthought in healthcare organizations, just as in any other organization. As I mentioned in the prologue, healthcare employees are notoriously unhealthy people. Though we know firsthand the effects of living an unhealthy lifestyle, personal motivation is still hard to come by.

We have discovered that a wellness program has motivation built into it, so employees don't have to conjure it on their own. If your wellness program is built out effectively, employees will be motivated to make changes without your having to force anybody to do anything.

THE BENEFITS

The first—and most obvious—benefit of an employee

wellness program is better health for all involved. Many of our employees have undergone incredible transformations. Some have lost a significant amount of weight. Others have been motivated to participate in local races. A few have even seen chronic diseases alleviated, or they have completely eliminated their need for medications.

When one person betters their health, others around them are affected. For example, when one person in a family starts to eat differently, the rest of the family will also make changes in their diet. When you consider your organization from a wider perspective, this effect on the families of employees is incredibly important, especially if you're insuring the spouse and the kids. When family members are constantly sick, on medications, or undergoing procedures, the cost of insurance can get out of hand.

Working in healthcare, I am fortunate that about 80 percent of my workforce is female. In the home, the mother or wife is often the head of the household in terms of dictating what the family is eating. Essentially, she dictates the healthcare of the family. If the mother or wife is saying, "Okay, we're going to start eating a little differently," then that is what the family does. When we can inspire our predominantly female workforce, they in turn drive healthier outcomes in their families.

This is not to say that a wellness program will only be

effective for a female workforce. You just need to keep in mind that men are generally slower to adopt lifestyle changes, especially if their wife is not on board. Culturally speaking, men are often seen as more manly when they eat a lot of meat and a generally unhealthy diet. If your workforce is mostly male, you may encounter a few extra obstacles. This is where the right education comes in. We have seen men in our workplace become so inspired by what they learn that they're able to motivate their spouse to get educated as well. It all starts with a spark in one person who is willing to change. Their motivation will become contagious.

Beyond the obvious health benefits, a wellness program will result in cost savings in your company. Reduction in costs comes in a few different forms. First, employees are going to feel better and have more energy as they get healthier. They will be more productive in their day-to-day work, accomplishing more in less time. This leads to a cost reduction in the long term. In some cases, we found that our employees were productive enough that we could hire fewer people for a department than we had in the past.

As mentioned already, you will also save money by reducing costs related to health insurance. When you are insuring a healthier population, the rates go down significantly. When employees are healthier, they will go to the doctor less frequently, require fewer medications, and have fewer major surgeries and hospitalizations.

The cost of healthcare in the United States is now 17 percent of the US gross domestic product, and it is rising dramatically year after year—with no end in sight. Between Medicare and Medicaid, taxpayers are paying over a trillion dollars in healthcare costs. Corporations and employers continue to bear a large brunt of these rising healthcare costs, in part because their workforce is becoming sicker, especially as they age. Right now, we have a large baby boomer workforce in the United States, to the tune of over 80 million people who are reaching retirement age and are very sick. Many families are also living paycheck to paycheck, and one major healthcare event can bankrupt them. We hear these kinds of stories all the time.

Rising healthcare costs and an aging population of employees who often require above-average levels of care directly affect companies that provide insurance. Corporations across the country are seeing this single line item go up every year, and they often don't recognize the far-reaching effects a wellness program can have for them. Of course, your organization should provide an adequate safety net of insurance, but you can never go wrong by placing greater emphasis on prevention and healthy living in the first place, to decrease costs later down the road.

THE WIN-WIN

If executed correctly, an employee wellness program will be a win for employees and their families, which will therefore be a win for your company. Employees are more engaged when they know that the company they work for truly cares about them as people and isn't a faceless, nameless corporation. It makes all the difference when employees want to come to work because they feel supported.

We have seen our employees recover from chronic diseases and give all the thanks to their leaders and the organization for essentially saving their lives. You can't buy that type of commitment to an organization through any other means. Sure, you can motivate employees by increasing their pay, but that pales in comparison to the motivation that is driven out of a wellness program. If you invest in your employees and help them achieve their highest potential in terms of health, you will gain a priceless return on your investment. You can't buy loyalty, teamwork, and camaraderie in an organization, but these are all organic results that emerge from a well-delivered wellness program.

Ultimately, employee wellness programs are good for humanity. We must all learn to be more health conscious. Factory farming contributes to greenhouse gases, and the population of the United States is eating over a million chickens a day. If you consider the global population—seven billion right now and projected to be nine or ten billion by 2050—we simply cannot sustain our current trends. We need to be advocates for healthier eating and a healthier world. What is good for the employees at your organization will be good for the country and good for our planet.

At the end of the day, the most important things in life are family and health. I might go so far as to say health comes first because, if you don't have your health, then you won't have your family. I believe we win when we help a whole group of people recognize health as a number-one priority and then act accordingly.

WHAT TO EXPECT

Each chapter in this book focuses on a key point to consider as you develop your wellness program. Chapter 1 begins with an encouragement to start with you. No one around you is going to change unless you are first a role model for healthy living.

In chapter 2, we'll consider how to get leaders in your organization involved, buying into the movement you are building. Then, we'll consider how to cultivate a movement that is self-perpetuating in chapter 3. Once you have gotten everyone's attention, you will want to know how to educate your employees. That's what we'll focus on in chapter 4.

Chapter 5 focuses on food; when it comes to health and wellness, food should be a top consideration. Chapter 6 outlines incentives; using the right incentives will give your employees that extra little bit of motivation to try something new. Chapter 7 focuses on community; once you gain advocates within the community, then the movement really begins to grow. We'll also consider metrics in chapter 8. You can use metrics to create better targets and priorities.

We'll conclude by considering the future of health and healthcare and where we are headed as a country. Despite the disheartening facts about rising healthcare costs, we live in an exciting time for change. There is a huge movement happening right now in relation to health and food. People want to lose weight, get healthy, and feel better. Our country is at an exciting tipping point, and now is the perfect time for you to start a wellness program.

By the end of the book, you will be well equipped with the tools and understanding for launching, administering, and maintaining an employee wellness program. I will walk you through each step, sharing our organization's personal trials and errors along the way so that you can get a behind-the-scenes look at the process.

Let's begin by talking about you!

CHAPTER 1

IT STARTS WITH YOU

In order to help others, you have to start right where you are sitting, with your own motivation. Yes, this book is ultimately about creating a wellness program for a large group of people, but if you don't help yourself first, you won't be of service to anyone. You need to become the go-to person for questions about wellness, and this won't happen unless you are pursuing a healthy lifestyle and walking the walk every day.

Starting with you means taking charge of your own health. No one else can do this for you. In fact, most of the voices around you are telling you to go the other direction, to ignore the effects of unhealthy living. You will need determination, especially in the area of food.

Before we move any further, know that you can do this. You can eat a healthier diet. You can maintain a healthier lifestyle. Others have gone before you and achieved phenomenal results. I am just a normal guy, rank and file like anyone else, and I was able to achieve excellent results. I simply had to commit to the journey of healthy living, and I am calling you to do the same.

CALLING ALL LEADERS

If you are the CEO or top leader in your organization, you do not have an excuse to be unhealthy. Yes, you are busy. In fact, you are likely chronically stressed. However, this is an even bigger reason to live a healthy lifestyle and eat a healthy diet. We are stressed at work, doing our best to do a great job. We are stressed at home with responsibilities, kids, and bills. We are stressed about money. In the middle of all of this, we're stuck in traffic, breathing contaminated air, and subject to pollution and all the other environmental toxins affecting our body on a daily basis. Everyone is busy, but if you make time to get healthy, you'll have more energy. As a result, you will be able to be awake and productive for more hours each day.

I remember one leader in my organization who was constantly stressed out. He was often late and always tired. He was notorious for falling asleep in meetings after lunch. About two years into my role, he began asking me questions about my energy level, what I did to exercise, and what I did for my diet. I had a hard time believing this leader was a candidate for change, but I obliged him by answering his questions. When he saw I was willing to help him, he asked for even more information and a roadmap to success.

At the beginning of the next calendar year, he told me his New Year's resolution was to get healthy, lose weight, and get his blood pressure and cholesterol under control. On January 1, he went cold turkey, eliminating processed food and dairy from his diet. He started working out, getting up early to run, eating more fruits and vegetables, and meditating. In five months, he met his goals and was a picture of health for others. He dropped forty pounds and today runs marathons for fun. He rarely misses a workout and knows he doesn't feel his best when he does.

I would not have been able to predict that this person would have gone through such a major transformation, but I have learned that everyone makes the decision to change in their own time and for different reasons. Some people just get sick of feeling lousy, addicted to caffeine and never truly awake. For many, those extra pounds get old until they finally decide enough is enough. You have to figure out your *why*. Why are you making a change? What are the sacrifices and benefits involved? No one can change your life for you.

The status quo is to say, "I'm too busy. I'm too stressed. I can't make time for a healthier lifestyle." I challenge you to think oppositely. Because you are busy and stressed, you need to monitor your food intake, your stress level, and your overall lifestyle even more. If you don't, everyone will suffer. You, your family, and your employees alike.

I'm not here to tell you that making a life change is easy. You will have to rearrange your schedule and your family's schedule. You will have to more proactively plan your meals and make time to work out or get outside. It will be difficult. It will take sacrifice. But that's why it will change your life for the better.

Most employees are especially nervous about making changes to their diet. They have eaten the same food every day for years. They have cereal for breakfast, a sandwich for lunch, perhaps a quick, fast-food meal for dinner. To venture out to anything outside of the routine can be scary. Thinking hard about food and investing time in the area of diet is going against the cultural tendency toward choosing fast food. For all of these reasons, employees need you. They need a leader who has faced these same thoughts and fears and successfully moved past them.

QUESTIONS OF TIME AND MONEY

If you feel that you just don't have enough time to eat

healthier, let me encourage you that you do. I have a wife and two small kids. I am a leader in my organization. Still, I have been able to maintain a healthy diet. In fact, going back to eating the basics—vegetables, rice and beans, whole grains, fruits, wraps, smoothies, and salads—can save you time. You will not have to think as much about what you are going to eat.

You can save time whether you want your food to be made for you or you want to make it yourself. Even if you are not in a city, you likely have access to numerous healthy choices within a short drive. If you make your own food, you can learn to prepare healthy meals quickly. You can even take advantage of companies that will ship you plant-based recipes with all the ingredients. These meals can be prepared in thirty minutes or less. They are healthy, tasty, and cost-effective. Again, you have no excuse when it comes to time.

You might also worry that having a healthier diet requires spending more money. Let me again encourage you; I have not found this to be true. Instead, I have found many inexpensive, healthy food options, and my grocery bill has not gone up. Yes, you might spend a bit more time shopping for the right food, but the minimal extra effort is worth it in the long run. Remember: your health should be your top priority.

BE THE LIGHTHOUSE

Once, while listening to a podcast, I heard an analogy of a lighthouse that resonated with me. Captains or seamen on a boat look to a lighthouse as a guiding light. The lighthouse remains planted in place, and people only come to it when they are ready.

I advocate this kind of pull strategy, not a push strategy; and it is incredibly effective if you are willing to have commitment and patience. Just as you can't push people to a lighthouse if they don't want to go, you can't push people to make lifestyle changes if they are not ready. However, if you stay planted and committed, sooner or later, others will show up because of your light. You will be exactly the resource they need at some point along their journey.

The first step to being a lighthouse—a light for others—is to be well informed about food.

CREATE YOUR NUTRITION PLAN

I don't espouse any single, rigid diet, but I do subscribe to some basic principles when it comes to food. I recommend a plant-based, whole-food approach. The basic tenet of a plant-based, whole-food diet is to avoid any food that is processed, high in sugar, or made from dairy or animal protein. Many diets fit within this category, and the purpose of this book is not to debate which is best.

When you commit to making a plan and eating healthier, you will benefit in ways you never imagined. For example, I have enjoyed being able to get back into the kitchen and spend more time with my wife and kids as we learn about food together. This time together is extremely rewarding on multiple levels. Not only can you spend more time with your family, but you can also teach your kids about where food comes from and how it's grown. You can teach them how to get back to the basics, a skill that has largely been lost in our society.

EAT MORE SIMPLY

One way to understand simple eating is to examine people's diets in other countries. Interestingly, people in many other nations eat simple meals. This past year, I went to Cuba and Iceland. I was amazed at how fresh and full of flavor the food was in both countries. Of course, there's a reason for this. These countries grow all of their own food. They import only what they cannot grow. They fish locally and eat only what they catch.

My in-laws recently returned from an extended trip to Italy. They reported a similar experience to my own—explaining how the food was very simple and had so much flavor and taste. The food did not have all of the additives, salt, and sugar. Everything was grown naturally. In the United States, we do not eat this way anymore. Everything has a laundry list of ingredients.

Another way to understand how to eat more simply is to consider what people ate in the fifties. Likely, they ate very simply. During that time, it was normal for a whole family to share a four-ounce piece of meat. Everyone got a taste, but meat was not a major part of a person's diet. Today, because we are not eating simply, our health is suffering.

When the unhealthy food options we have created move into other nations, we see how connected food is to health. For example, the predominant foods in Asian countries have been rice and vegetables for hundreds of years. When fast-food restaurants were introduced in cities in Japan and China, the health of those populations almost immediately declined.

If you don't want to spend a lot of time researching nutrition, simply remember to avoid processed foods, animal protein, and dairy. Anything that is processed is not in its natural form and is often full of sugar. Too much animal protein can clog the vascular system. We often ignore the negative effects of dairy because we don't want to think about giving up our yogurt, ice cream, and cheese. However, we are the only animal on the planet that consumes another animal's milk—milk that is meant for a baby cow to grow. If you're interested in learning more about dairy in particular, I recommend *The Cheese Trap* by Dr. Neal Barnard. He talks about how cheese lights up the same dopamine receptors in our brains as heroin does, which makes it an incredibly addictive food. He also speaks about how it causes inflammation, mucus, and general stress on the body.

If you are the researching type, there are endless resources available to dive deep into the topic of healthy eating and how to make positive changes in your diet. A couple of thought leaders in particular have influenced my own thinking. Many of them have come to give talks at our hospital, and their message has been highly impactful for many employees. Brendan Brazier, who wrote *Thrive*, is one of these thought leaders. Another is Dr. Caldwell Esselstyn from the Cleveland Clinic. Dr. Michael Greger has an amazing website with a ton of resources, and Dr. Neal Barnard has written a number of books that focus on diet. Most recently, I have been enjoying learning from Dr. Doug Graham, who focuses on the importance of fruit in the human diet.

UNDERSTAND WHERE EXERCISE FITS

I place an emphasis on food—even over exercise—because what you eat has greater influence over your health than how you exercise. Exercise is important, but it's hard to exercise your way out of an unhealthy body if you are eating poorly. See the prologue for my personal experience with this reality. If you are not eating a healthy diet, it doesn't matter how hard you exercise; you will likely still gain weight.

In order to thrive and have a long life, you need to move your body. That's a given. However, even seemingly fit athletes have heart attacks and strokes. They don't look unhealthy, but they are. Many bodybuilders and wrestlers look like they are in amazing shape, for example, but they're eating a diet heavy in animal protein and clogging up their vascular systems. We see the devastating results on the news all the time.

If you are new to exercise or think you are doing it wrong, I suggest you seek out a personal trainer or someone certified to train. There are also tons of resources online, including online coaching. Find someone who is able to prescribe workouts based on your skill level and abilities. Always start slow and understand your limits. You don't want to do a marathon on day one. Whatever exercise you decide to do to get your body moving and your heart rate up, remember that the best regimen will incorporate both cardiovascular workouts and some resistance training. Resistance training is especially important for longevity and healthy muscles and bones.

When it comes to exercise, remember to pick something that you enjoy doing, and you'll be more inclined to stick with it. You can also set goals for yourself and work out with a buddy or group of friends. When you have fitness goals that you need to meet or other people whom you are accountable to, you will be much more likely to stick with your 5:00 a.m. wakeup time to work out. Otherwise, it is too easy to hit the snooze button and go back to sleep.

So yes, exercise is important, but even more important is to be aware of what is going on inside of your body. When you eat high-calorie, high-sugar, and highly processed foods, your leptin or insulin responses are not communicating to your brain that you need to get out and move. You're getting dopamine hits from the foods you're eating, and you just want to sit on the couch and eat more sugary, highly processed food. They make your brain feel good, but not your body. Eating poorly brings you back to square one—with no motivation to exercise.

Contrast this with eating a healthy diet. When you start consuming more nutritious food, your brain realizes that your body is getting the fuel it needs to exercise. In this way, diet and exercise work hand in hand.

DON'T IGNORE THE INDUSTRIAL FOOD COMPLEX

Today, only a handful of food companies control most of the food distribution in the country. Food has become big business, and you can't necessarily fault these companies or their leaders. Many of them are public companies, so they're incentivized to make a profit. Wall Street is watching their stocks. However, we have to recognize that their main goal of turning a profit has been to the detriment of our citizens and our health as a nation.

The food industry pushes out heavily processed foods every day. These foods are usually high in sodium and some type of sugar, whether high-fructose corn syrup or a sugar alternative. These foods also have a high number of ingredients and are the opposite of simple food. Many large food companies have scientists in labs scientifically enhancing the ingredients in foods so that they will light up certain pleasure parts of our brains. The goal is to make our brains say, "Wow, this food is great! I want more."

Several recent studies have compared eating one meal from a standard American diet (SAD) with smoking half a pack of cigarettes. In other words, in terms of carcinogens and toxins, the food we are eating is having the same kind of effect on the body as smoking.

When tobacco companies were trying hard to hold their market share, they first denied that smoking was actually bad for you. Later, they created studies that raised confusion in the public. People would wonder: *Is smoking actually bad for us?* No one knew what to believe. The same sense of confusion now exists in our nation around food. People are now wondering: *Is my diet actually unhealthy? What is actually contributing to disease? What should the food pyramid actually look like?* It's difficult for consumers to know what direction to take.

The food industry has become extremely efficient in providing unhealthy food to the public, all at an appealing cost. Farms are built to push out high volumes—especially with corn, soy, and animal products. Animals are grown to unnatural sizes, and their feed is filled with antibiotics, steroids, and hormones. Likely, you have seen one or two documentaries that have brought some light to this new phenomenon of efficient, but unhealthy ways of providing food to the population. Consumers continue to demand these foods, however, and the demand creates an endless cycle. In the United States, we kill approximately one million animals every ninety minutes to satisfy the huge demand for animal products. This is not sustainable.

With two-thirds of our population now overweight, we know that something is clearly wrong. The movement toward healthier eating is now being led by some amazing thought leaders who are helping to educate the public. Nonetheless, until the movement's message creates change in the food on your own table, it remains little more than a nice idea.

As you consider how to start with yourself and how to be a guiding light for others, remember that we all vote with our money every day. Healthier options continue to be made more readily available as more people demand them. You can demand healthier options, and you can encourage a whole group of people to do the same.

STARTING WITH ME

Before I considered helping develop our employee wellness program, I had my own journey with food. As mentioned in the prologue, my life filled up with many stressors at once. My wife and I moved, I started a new job, and my parents were both diagnosed with chronic diseases. I was gaining a lot of weight no matter how much I worked out, and I knew something needed to change. I finally made a decision to be more proactive about my health.

I began to dive into research and decided to follow everything Brendan Brazier recommended in *Thrive*. After only a month of my commitment to change, I had more energy, was sleeping better, and simply felt better. I remember noticing how, for the first time, I felt great while driving in to work—fully ready for the day.

As the leader of an organization, I naturally wanted to spread the knowledge I had gained and encourage my team to live healthier lives and to experience the benefits I was experiencing. I wanted the people I worked side by side with every day to feel as great as I did, so I began thinking about how we could improve our employee wellness program using the pull strategy.

THE IMPORTANCE OF YOUR STORY

Over time, I noticed that others who had made changes and had seen positive results in their health had the same desire as I had to spread the word and help others. No one was being forceful and saying, "Watch your weight. You have to work out." We were simply a group of people with powerful stories. True momentum toward healthy living requires this community of stories, and it starts with yours.

When you are willing to share your story without any expectations, other people will be drawn by your light. When employees can talk with someone who is a "normal" person and has had success, they can start to believe that making changes could work for them too. You don't have to be on a soapbox saying, "Go do this." You just have to be an inspirational role model, and people will automatically be drawn to you. Conversations will happen naturally, and you will have opportunities to recommend tools or steps that have worked for you.

We live in a world where it's hard to know where to turn and what information to trust. I read a stat recently that said only one-tenth of 1 percent of the population is able to lose weight and keep it off. The weight-loss programs out there are ineffective, and people are constantly moving up and down without lasting results. Naturally, people become skeptical over time about any new "program." However, if your wellness program focuses on people's real stories—how someone has lost weight or overcome a chronic disease—people will start listening.

One employee, whom we'll call George, had one of those inspirational stories. George was overweight and had been for a long time. He couldn't run, because his knees could not take the pounding, so he started swimming and biking instead. Over the course of a year, he changed his diet and logged mile after mile in the water and on the bike. Initially, he couldn't swim or bike quickly, but he was nevertheless burning a lot of calories. Soon enough, everything about him began to change. He was happier, had more energy, and was sleeping better. His digestive system was working better, and the pounds melted off. After a year, George was at his target weight.

Whenever someone can lose a significant amount of weight and keep it off, we are all impressed. With the kind of food that surrounds us, this can be a difficult task. Because George's struggle with his weight was so familiar to others, I began to send employees to hear his story. He would tell them how he only saw results when he acknowledged that a quick fix would not work. The weight was never going to come off with a crash diet or gimmick from an infomercial. He would explain how he put on the weight over many years, and it was never going to come off in a week or a month. Results required day-to-day discipline. Today, George continues to inspire others as a living example of someone who achieved his goals and can now thrive, instead of struggle.

FIND YOUR *WHY*

Everyone wants to feel better. Everyone wants to live a long and healthy life. No one wants to take twelve pills a day or have trouble sleeping. Every person, however, has a different *why*.

As you consider how to start with you, I encourage you to think about your own *why*. Maybe you want to lose ten pounds to run a marathon and feel better. Maybe you want to be a good role model for your kids and be able to play with your grandkids on the floor when you're seventy-five. Maybe you want to be able to travel in your golden years without needing a wheelchair or oxygen.

When you're thinking about your *why*, consider both the present and the future. Yes, your present goal should be to wake up every day feeling good and ready for the day. It's important, however, to consider the rest of your life as well. The status quo says, "It's normal to get a chronic disease or generally struggle as you age." You might be prone to think: *I have heart disease in my family, so it's part of my genetics. I'm just waiting to have a heart attack.* However, you have a choice about how you shape your health. You have the choice to embrace a bigger purpose and see your life from a wider perspective.

What do you want your later years to look like? What do you want them to look like for your employees?

In my line of work, I'm often saddened to see people who have been saving for retirement their whole lives only to have a major health event and have to come into the hospital. They become debilitated or are simply unable to thrive anymore. I hate seeing these people in and out of the hospital, having numerous surgeries, taking a lot of pills, and generally not feeling well. On the other end of the spectrum, I have seen people thrive well into their eighties and nineties. When I recently participated in a local triathlon, there were two eighty-year-olds who were also there. They looked great and did well in the race, and I fully believe that everyone can follow in their footsteps.

The first step is to find your *why*. Knowing your greater purpose will motivate you to make health a priority, and your priorities will dictate your decisions. By making health a priority, you can have more energy in life now and enjoy your later years as well.

My hope is that this chapter has inspired you to think about your own health journey and the ways in which your proactive approach toward wellness will directly affect others in your organization. Now it's time to turn your attention outward—toward other leaders around you. Their buy-in is essential for the success of the wellness program, but gaining their support is not always easy. In the next chapter, I will outline ways that you can effectively approach leaders and help them see the value of your new mission.

CHAPTER 2

BUY-IN FROM LEADERS

Everyone in an organization can influence the success of a wellness program. Employees who are living and promoting healthy lifestyles will propel wellness initiatives forward. However, if you don't have buy-in from leaders at the top of your organization, you will have a difficult time getting a wellness program off the ground in the first place. Even if you are able to launch a program, significant long-term results won't be what they could have been without other leaders' support. I have seen many wellness programs without full leadership support end up being "flavor-of-the-month" programs without a long-term vision. A few people in the company will participate each month, but the company will never be able to build a culture that moves toward wellness.

When leaders are involved, especially high-level leaders, you have a greater chance of creating a holistic wellness program that effects change. Leadership involvement not only will result in a stronger vision for the program, but it will also show that those at the top truly care about each employee. In my leadership role, I have recognized that employees want to feel not only that they are adding value to the company, but also that they are appreciated as individuals with full lives. Within that full life of each employee, there's not a conversation more important than one about health. Offering a workplace wellness program communicates to an employee that the company leadership cares about their health and well-being—that the leadership is willing to invest in them and their families.

What other leaders in your company need to understand is that their buy-in will result in a return on investment. When an employee feels cared for, they are more loyal to the company and its leadership. As they are more loyal, they are then more productive. Younger generations of employees especially value being part of a team, and they will not give blind loyalty to any organization. They have to first know that the leaders representing the organization care about them.

One important point to keep in mind here is that it isn't imperative to have buy-in from every top leader. That said, you need at least one person in the executive suite who is clearly on board and will champion the effort. Of course, the more buy-in you get, the better.

You also want to seek buy-in from middle management—the directors, managers, and supervisors who are working "in the trenches" on a day-to-day basis. If these leaders, who are often the most visible to employees, model healthy living with good behaviors and choices, then their employees will see that and feel empowered to ask them about their lifestyles and experiences. Middle management can then communicate with the top-level leaders, especially the one senior leader who is clearly on board with worksite wellness. When you get to the point where different levels of leadership are communicating specifically about wellness to employees, you will begin to see greater progress in every area of the program—from financial support to lives being changed.

THE DANGER OF LUKEWARM SUPPORT

Historically, there has been lip service paid to prevention of illness and employee wellness. Healthcare has always been an expense for companies, and yet that line item continues to grow. The issue has grown large enough that everyone is now starting to pay attention, wondering how to trim that cost. If there are not major changes in employee health and wellness, nothing will change; that is the hard truth. If we keep doing what we're doing, the costs will continue to rise, and employees will continue to lead unhealthy lifestyles, suffer chronic disease, and be negatively affected in their work and home life.

For this reason, lukewarm support from leaders is simply not an option. If you don't have buy-in at every level of leadership, the program simply won't work and the health-care line item will not decrease. Without strong C-suite and middle management support, you will only be able to capture the attention of employees who were already predisposed to caring about wellness. If you want to achieve company-wide change, lukewarm support from your leaders will not do.

An example of lukewarm support is when a leader says all the right things in meetings, but their actions are counter to the promotion of health and wellness. In public, everyone typically agrees that wellness and prevention are important. Still, unless the majority of your leaders are truly bought in, your initiatives will not reach their full potential.

When you have strong leadership support on every level, employees will feel comfortable discussing the wellness programs and opportunities for wellness. They will feel empowered to have a voice. Not all employees would be comfortable going to the CEO or the chief human resources officer to talk about their health. They may be willing, however, to talk to their immediate supervisor who is modeling healthy living. On the other hand, middle managers need to have a voice as well. They need someone above them to listen to their ideas.

In our organization, gaining leadership buy-in at every level took time, but ultimately we were able to have support at several levels. These leaders showed their support by participating. They changed their diets and their workout routines. They paid attention to their mental health by incorporating activities such as meditation and yoga. They had fantastic lab results, and many lost a lot of weight. They became role models, and many of them were willing to share their stories. Every company needs these leaders—those who are willing to help employees on their personal journeys toward wellness by providing positive feedback, tools, and resources.

As leaders move beyond lukewarm support to full buy-in, every level of the organization is affected. Ultimately, employees should have access to many points of inspiration, rather than only a couple of high-level leaders whose stories aren't getting out.

OUR EXAMPLE

As a top-level leader of our hospital, I had the advantage of being able to disperse information about wellness to the entire company. When we first started to focus more on the wellness program, I decided I needed to be a role model. I led a healthy lifestyle and tried to be as approachable as possible when any other leader or employee wanted to ask me about my focus on wellness. I would send out articles for employees to read if they wanted, and I also asked for feedback on what we could do to continue to invest in our employees, especially in their health and wellness. As our program grew, I gave employees books and documentaries to help them become educated about health and wellness and the changes they could make in their lives.

Employee response to my leadership in wellness was mixed. Employees would often stop me in the hallway and ask why we were focusing on health and why the food being offered in the cafeteria was changing. I remember one doctor demanding we put the fryers back in the cafeteria, so he could continue to eat his fried foods when he came to the hospital. Some employees were excited and jumped in right away. Some wanted to wait and see what their colleagues and leaders did before committing. Others were reluctant to change at all. We didn't focus on the latter group, but continued to offer them education and encouraged them to talk to their colleagues who had experienced success. Many of them started to realize that they, too, could experience success in getting healthier.

Beyond providing employees with educational resources and programs, I focused on initiating conversations. My aim as a leader was to get ideas for what we could do differently and take that feedback and create opportunities for health and wellness. Instead of taking things away, I created new offerings based on employee feedback. I wanted to create an environment where anyone could seek me out and ask questions. I wanted to be the example of the lighthouse. As I did this, other leaders started getting excited about sharing their own stories and successes. When an employee would approach me, I would sometimes offer resources or encouragement directly, but I would often redirect them to another leader or employee in the organization who had had success. This way, conversations became less forced.

OBSTACLES TO BUY-IN

Many people assume that because I led a healthcare organization, it was easy for me to get other leaders to participate in worksite wellness. That wasn't necessarily the case.

In the early stages, I made sure the internal discussion revolved around holistic approaches to wellness, ones that ensured that mind, body, and spirit were in alignment. I made sure to offer several programs to our leaders. One was called "Natural Leadership," which was given by

consultants who talked about mindfulness and meditation. Still, gaining buy-in from other leaders was not easy.

MOTIVATION

In general, healthcare workers are not the healthiest group
of people. There is always a lot of unhealthy food, like
donuts, available in hospitals. Everyone is also always on
the go, grabbing food on the run. Some leaders struggled
to have motivation to change their lifestyles because they
saw doctors and nurses fix people every day. If a patient
had a heart attack or a stroke, the doctors or surgeons
could fix them. When you live in that world for too long,
you start to assume that chronic disease can be fixed very
easily. When you know there is a backup and safety net
called "the hospital," it can be difficult to motivate yourself to change your habits and get healthier on your own.
Healthcare workers got into the profession because they
wanted to help others, but they tend to neglect themselves
a little bit more than the average person. We want to give
our all to others, at the expense of ourselves. Our health is
one of the first things to go, if we don't pay attention to it.

While all of these problems seem unique to the healthcare industry, they are not. In general, leaders tend to
be busy and are concerned about getting things done or
about taking care of people and making sure everything
is running smoothly. Nowadays, leaders have a difficult

time turning off their jobs. They're checking emails in the evening and all weekend. Work is on their smartphone, and it's all too easy to stay connected. There's always something a leader can be doing, and they often end up feeling as if they are working twenty-four hours a day, seven days a week. Leaders are on more than they're off, and they're not getting a mental break. Ultimately, leadership buy-in for a wellness program can become difficult because leaders simply feel they don't have enough time. Of course, the high-stress lifestyle they lead is exactly why they need to focus on their health.

CHANGE IS NOT EASY

Another major obstacle to leadership buy-in is people's stubbornness to change. Most people, including leaders, like their routines. For example, they have eaten the same type of food every day for a long time, and they like it that way. Some need for change goes unrecognized. Most modern-day workers, employees and leaders alike, sit at their desk all day long. Unless there is a designated time for employees to get up and move, they won't. This is why adding rather than subtracting is important in implementing a wellness program. In our organization, we started offering new food in the cafeteria rather than taking items away so that change would not seem negative and become an obstacle.

Older, more established corporations will be the slowest

to change. Typically, the problem starts with the leaders' hesitancy to change. Today, we're seeing younger organizations with younger leaders valuing employees a bit more from the start. They're creating wellness programs and focusing on investing in their people. Yet, with the growing cost of healthcare, leaders at every organization, no matter how old it is, are paying more attention. The problem is that few leaders have any idea where to begin.

THE COST CONCERN

Many leaders make money an obstacle to wellness, which is often just an excuse. It may seem that changing your diet, starting to work out, and concentrating more on your health would increase personal expenses. However, the real question is where you want to spend your dollars. When leaders are hesitant to invest in their own health, I always try to help them see the bigger picture. I take them back to the beginning: if you don't have your health, you don't have anything. Some leaders take time to consider this reality and begin to make changes little by little. Others will sit back to wait and see how things work out with others around them who have chosen to change.

Within your own business, creating a wellness program for employees will have a cost associated with it. Many leaders have a hard time seeing past this initial reality. If they could look past the dollars needed in the budget to fund a wellness program, they would recognize the payoff on the back end. Ultimately, a wellness program will result in cost savings because the company will have healthier employees. As you consider leaders in your own company, think about which ones might be able to see the value of spending money upfront for long-term results.

STORIES THAT MULTIPLY BUY-IN

If you are still feeling uneasy about getting buy-in from top executives at your organization, I want to encourage you. You might know your company absolutely must start focusing more on the health of employees. You might understand that change starts with you. Even so, you might not feel that any other leaders are willing to join the efforts with you. I want to encourage you that leadership buy-in often develops as stories multiply. If you and perhaps one other leader have stories to share about what wellness has meant to you, then you can move the ball forward.

Whenever you find genuine enthusiasm from top leaders, be sure to spread that enthusiasm to others. This will help you paint worksite wellness in a positive light. Talk about positive changes you have seen in your life and the lives of other leaders who have bought in to living healthy lifestyles during every opportunity you have—whether via email, in newsletters, or at meetings. Optimism spreads quickly; it's contagious. If you and your company's leaders are excited about creating a healthier employee population, other leaders, and ultimately employees, will buy in and be more likely to try new things.

Leaders who have bought in will also be effective in connecting employees to each other. Certain pockets of employees will be early adopters. They will have quick success and see their health improve dramatically, in a short period of time. Some of them will be outspoken and willing to share their stories. Leaders should know who these people are.

Other employees will be more quietly making changes behind the scenes. You will see them a month later, and they will seem like completely different people. These people will also become role models, but rather than being outspoken like the first group, they will come out of the woodwork to tell their stories. Their experiences will lead to a groundswell of support for whatever health and wellness program you've launched.

We had one employee with debilitating rheumatoid arthritis in her hands and joints. She was always uncomfortable and had a lot of swelling and inflammation. I saw her in the cafeteria one day and started a conversation. I asked her how she was doing, and she admitted she wasn't feeling well. She told me the swelling had been going on for a year or two and that she was on several medications.

As a leader, I focused on knowing the stories of success throughout the company. I immediately thought of someone to connect her with, who had beaten cancer through lifestyle changes. They talked, and she made some changes in her diet and lifestyle. She switched to a whole-food, plant-based diet and started meditating. Six weeks later, she had almost totally healed her rheumatoid arthritis. She was in no way upset that I had connected her with another employee. Instead, she was incredibly thankful to learn from someone else who had been on a similar journey. The employee she spoke with had essentially healed himself, and so did she. This was a perfect example of the power of stories. Stories need to start with leaders, but they don't stop there.

Stories spread like wildfire throughout an organization. Others hear them and want to know more. The optimism and positivity are exciting. This creates a great foundation for later stages of worksite wellness. Buy-in from the top, without having a way to ensure the stories are out in the open, does not allow the positivity to spread. Employees need to know exactly where to go when they are ready to ask questions, whether that is to a leader or to another employee a leader connects them with.

VALUE IN PERSEVERING

Keep in mind that buy-in from leadership is a gradual

process. It does not happen overnight. Anytime you talk with someone about their health, it's very personal. You must move slowly with any changes in this area.

I encourage companies to create two-year to four-year plans and lay out what will happen at every stage. I advocate for small changes because this is how you will realistically get buy-in at every level of the company. If you try to do everything at once, people will be shocked. They will push back and likely react negatively to the program. If you focus on small changes over time, you are saying to leaders that you value their involvement in the process, without forcing them to do anything. You can start with minor adjustments in the cafeteria. One month, you might start offering milk alternatives (almond and soy). Another month, you might offer baked potatoes instead of french fries. As you go, you can ask leaders how they feel about the changes and communicate clearly that you care about their input.

Don't forget to educate leaders as you make changes. They, after all, will be the spokespeople for the wellness program. You have probably heard the story of the frog in boiling water. If you put a frog in cold water and slowly turn the heat up, they don't jump out. However, if you put a frog in boiling water, it will jump out. It's the same with people concerning their health and wellness. They are much more likely to accept subtle, small changes over time (two, three, or four years) without jumping out of the water. They will stick with you, ask questions, and continue to work on their own health along the way.

When you get leadership buy-in, you are set up for a true movement, which we will explore in the next chapter. Having multiple leaders involved means that a company is valuing employees, not viewing them as another cog in the machine. I am reminded of being a platoon leader in the Army, in charge of thirty-eight soldiers. I wasn't just in charge of them from 6:00 a.m. to 6:00 p.m. I felt a sense of responsibility for everything in their lives—their families, their kids, their health, and sometimes even their finances. In the private sector, leaders are rarely that involved in their employees' lives. However, you have an opportunity to communicate to your whole organization that the leaders do care. I am hopeful that more and more leaders will recognize the importance of health not only in their own lives but in the lives of their employees as well.

CHAPTER 3

LAUNCHING A MOVEMENT

Once you gain buy-in from leaders and others within your organization, communication should accelerate. You can start by sending messages using different mediums about some additional offerings. Next, you will want to consider how to share some of the success stories. The key is to get the word out, inviting people by simply saying, "Here's what we're doing."

MESSAGING

So what does the messaging look like? First, you should always aim to make it positive, with an inviting tone. You should also make sure the communication recognizes the whole person; it needs to come from a place of caring.

With each message, you are telling your employees that you care about them and also their families. You don't want to communicate that you are forcing them to do anything. Simply say, "We're providing more resources, tools, and opportunities for you to get educated, get healthy, and change your lifestyle. How you participate is up to you."

Your messaging should be inclusive, encouraging, and nonjudgmental. You could communicate through email, newsletters, department meetings, or town hall meetings. I remember one particular email that I wrote around the holidays one year. I emphasized that everyone takes time for themselves to recharge and to spend time with their families and loved ones. I explained that if we are not fully present at work, we cannot reach our potential. I was surprised by how many employees wrote me back and told me how much they appreciated that I cared about them getting some personal time. They appreciated that I made a point of taking care of their families and personal issues first. Many said they really felt cared for when they read that note. It was simple to send an email, but it meant a lot.

When you are communicating about new programs, make sure it is clear that anyone can participate. Sometimes, especially when it comes to diet and weight-related issues, people doubt their abilities. It is your job to help employees believe they can do it. Encourage them with uplifting words. Express clearly that the company cares and wants to invest in them. If the company believes they are worth it, they, in turn, will believe they are worth it.

Be clear that the company is not judging anyone on the failures they have had so far on their journey to health and wellness. You are providing tools and resources to help them find success. The majority of people don't know the best ways to eat, work out, or improve their mental health. Eating right, in particular, is tough; there's no doubt about that. Food is engineered these days to spark responses in the pleasure center of the brain. Inevitably, employees will feel sensitive when it comes to topics around health. Recognize that everyone is on a journey, and message accordingly.

GETTING EMPLOYEES INVOLVED

If employees are not getting involved, the movement won't go anywhere. This is why it is important to provide a lot of different opportunities for getting involved. You should have opportunities related to food, exercise, and mental health. When an employee experiences success in one area, they will be more willing to try something in another area. When people start working out, for example, they are more likely to want to eat healthier and consider their mental health. When people start eating healthier, they will feel better and want to work out. When people start meditating, their brains aren't as fuzzy and they'll have space and time to think. All three areas are connected.

If you can pull an employee into one of those areas, their success there will likely lead to participation in the other areas. Your goal, then, is to help everyone try at least one thing.

Hosting community events is one way to encourage people to get healthy. Your company could start by sponsoring a 5K, a triathlon, or a "Vegfest." Publicize the events to employees, and encourage them to participate. Once an employee begins participating and sees others participating as well, he or she will be more likely to continue. It's easier for anyone to be part of a community event than to do something on their own. People need to feel they are part of something bigger than themselves. As you sponsor local races or wellness events, be sure to get leaders involved. When employees see their leaders involved in these events, they want to get involved too.

A simple way to get employees involved in moving toward wellness is by being proactive and asking for employee discounts from gyms or wellness centers in your area. Discounts provide people with an incentive to exercise, and this might also build camaraderie and accountability as employees begin exercising together. You might also ask for discounts from healthier restaurants to funnel your employees there; this should be a win-win for your employees and the restaurants. An added benefit is that by supporting restaurants that offer healthy food, it will allow these restaurants to stay in business, and new healthier restaurants might spring up as well.

CHIP

At our organization, one of the ways we got employees involved was by offering CHIP, which stands for Complete Health Improvement Program. We sent messages, explaining it was completely optional, but we were offering it because we valued employees' health. CHIP is a national program that includes eighteen classes over the course of three months. Employees get divided into groups of eight to twenty, and the classes teach them about health and wellness, specifically around food. CHIP does have a cost (about $650), but it's an investment well worth the price tag. Early on, our health insurance didn't cover CHIP, so we offered to pay half of the cost for our employees to enroll in the program.

We've had fantastic success with this single program. It's medically managed, which means the people running it do labs and blood work at the beginning and throughout the program. At the end, employees can see the often-dramatic improvement in their labs and overall health. Their success encourages other employees to want to get involved.

COST CONSIDERATIONS

As you consider how to get employees involved, you will likely want to consider financial restraints. For example, if you want to get employees, as well as their spouses and families, involved, discounts to gyms or restaurants will rarely cost you anything. The CHIP program is a significant cost, but if one person in the family takes the program, they will learn the strategies for healthy eating and living and can then share that information with the rest of the family. Some spouses will choose to be involved in programs that do have a cost. The key, again, is to offer options. Employees and their families can choose how to interact with those options.

More and more insurance plans are offering full reimbursement for health education programs. They understand that healthier employees lead to fewer claims and less money they're paying out for healthcare bills. Spending $650 on the front end toward prevention and wellness is a smart investment for them. As you consider different programs, be sure to see what you can have covered through insurance. The more you can cover, the more options you can offer.

CHALLENGES TO THE MOVEMENT

Launching a movement starts with the right messaging and getting employees involved in as many ways as possible. It also requires planning. As mentioned, consider creating a two-year to four-year plan. On the front end of that plan, you will want to provide as many educational opportunities as you can. In addition, educational opportunities should be offered each year. As more employees get involved, promote different options, such as races, gym discounts, and contests.

As you launch this movement, expect the initial reaction to be mixed, from leaders and employees. Some people in your organization will buy in immediately. Some will wait and see. Some will be skeptical.

I remember one of our employees who came up to me after about a year on the job. She was happy I was making health and wellness a priority, but she was also hesitant to say the initiatives could benefit her. She felt she was genetically predisposed to being obese. Her parents were obese, her kids were obese, and she thought she was destined to be obese. I tried to encourage her by explaining the research I have read, which states that health and wellness is predominantly due to environment and that each person does have a choice. I gave her examples in our own organization of employees and patients who had success on the journey. I told her she was a fantastic employee (which she is) and that she could accomplish anything if she set her mind to it.

That little extra motivation from me lit a spark within her, and she committed to a healthier lifestyle. We agreed she would connect with me monthly and update me on her progress. Today, she is at her target weight, very active, and has a lot more energy. She committed to success and made it happen. She is a great reminder that the hesitation many people feel about getting healthier is not an impassable obstacle. Oftentimes, people need just a little motivation.

Still, you will always face challenges as the movement progresses. Every company has a lot going on, and people are busy. Leaders and employees may experience "initiative fatigue" when there are too many initiatives going on at once. However, initiative fatigue typically occurs when initiatives come and go each month. A wellness program is not the same; it's not going away. If you engrain wellness into the culture of your organization, it becomes "the way we do it here" rather than another initiative. One way to show the wellness program isn't going anywhere is by sharing your two-year to four-year plan with your employees, not just your leaders. This will help employees see how much you value wellness.

The culture that sets wellness as a top priority should be clearly communicating your care for employees. Every chance you get, remind them that you care about them. Yes, you want your employees to be highly productive, but you also want them to lead healthy, happy lives. For all of these reasons, you want to invest in their health.

SETTING EXPECTATIONS

As you see the movement begin, keep your expectations in check. At this point, you're still trying to build momentum, and that takes time. It also takes time for people to get healthier. If you are the type of leader or organization that has to see results in a month or two, this isn't for you. This is a long-term strategy. People's lives will change, but you have to be willing to be patient. Seeing results sometimes takes years.

Do your best not to get frustrated if you are not seeing the results you had hoped for in the early stages. Stay the course. Keep messaging. Keep inviting people to learn more. Keep providing opportunities to get involved. Stay positive and optimistic, and share the success stories. Stick to the plan. Eventually, you will reach a tipping point where the movement does become self-sustaining because enough people are noticing positive changes or have already experienced major breakthroughs. They're feeling better and looking better. They're excited about what they've accomplished. Not only do these successes equal a healthier workforce, but they equal a better company all around.

HOW MOVEMENTS HAPPEN

You may have seen that famous YouTube video that went viral a few years ago of a man at a concert. At first, he's dancing all alone; it's a strange dance with bizarre movements. Other people are sitting on the lawn watching him. Soon enough, a second person joins him, then a third, then three more people. Eventually, you see groups of five, ten, and fifteen people jump in until there's a giant crowd of people doing this weird dance, moving their bodies in hilarious ways.

This is how a movement happens. Everyone likes being part of a movement, but you need the trailblazers, the early adopters, and those who wait and see before joining in. If you want to know how a movement happens, watch that YouTube video.

One story comes to mind of an employee who was significantly overweight. I would share books and documentaries with him. He would never read the books, and he would only sometimes watch the documentaries. He'd say, "I don't know if I believe all that. I'm a meat eater, and I like meat. I want to keep eating meat." He wouldn't buy in to the suggestions I would throw his way. Then he had a heart attack, which put him in the hospital. That was his wake-up call.

Some of us focus on our health before we have a scare;

others wait until the scare happens. This employee got serious about his health. He went to the CHIP classes. He started eating a whole-food, plant-based diet. Ultimately, he lost a lot of weight and felt much better. His success story now helps others who say, "I don't know if I believe all that." He is a perfect resource for those who aren't the trailblazers or early adopters, but who stand back and wait. When they hear his story, they can't help but wonder if they should join the movement too. Many people are just stuck in the way they've always done things. They like their routines. They're not going to change until they hear a story that connects with them personally.

In many cases, we have seen employees finally get excited about joining the movement once they connect with the insight they didn't previously have. This is why educational opportunities are vital. We'll focus on the many ways you can educate your team in the next chapter.

CHAPTER 4

EDUCATING YOUR TEAM

Along the path to health, we must become more informed. Everyone inherently knows how important health is, but very few people think about it every day. Sometimes, we don't think about our health until we don't feel well or something bad happens to us. A strong wellness program should promote more regular thought and discussion around health.

You can help support this regular thought and discussion in your company by encouraging employees that there is always more to learn. As a leader who is invested in employees' health, you can provide that constant education. Healthy living is a lifelong journey. No one can learn everything there is to know in a month and then be done. So how, exactly, can you continually educate your team?

EDUCATIONAL OPPORTUNITIES

The more opportunities for education that you offer, the more quickly you will build interest in the wellness movement. Educational opportunities might look like exercise classes (yoga, aerobics, weight lifting) and meditation classes. You can subsidize these or bring them into the workplace to make it easy for employees to participate over lunch or before/after work. Another great way to promote education is by equipping leaders with resources—books, articles, or documentaries—that they can use for their own learning and also hand out to others. Everyone learns differently, so providing several different types of tools is a smart move.

You might also consider bringing in speakers from outside your organization. We had a very good response when we brought in national speakers and experts in the field. It's one thing to read someone's book, but it's another to have the author show up at your workplace, give a talk, and answer questions. That can stir a lot of excitement within the organization. People love hearing from experts and inspirational speakers, and every employee will connect with different speakers in different ways. Some employees have particular athletic goals and want to hear from athletes. Others want to lose weight and want to hear from doctors or people who have lost a lot of weight themselves. Inviting a variety of speakers allows a wide range of your employees to connect with the movement.

I already mentioned the CHIP program, but it's worth mentioning again. This program is not necessarily group therapy, but it is fun and provides accountability through group work. When employees know they will see their group within a few days, they'll be ready to talk about what they ate or if they cheated. There are different timeframes required for building different habits. In the area of food, the real scientists say it takes sixty days to change your diet, to get through detox, and to stop eating unhealthy fare. Because the CHIP program lasts several months, employees have the opportunity to go through those stages, and they will be with a group of people experiencing the same things. They can talk and relate. At the same time, they can become more informed about why the changes are important and what is going on in their bodies.

Through CHIP and similar programs, employees can learn healthy recipes in class and see cooking demonstrations. They learn how to cook and eat healthy food on the go and how to order healthy food at restaurants. In CHIP, participants get to cook for each other and eat together.

Health is not a topic that is widely discussed. It is considered a personal thing; every person deals with their own health by themselves. Unfortunately, this means that there is little understanding of how to talk about wellness with others. Without a way to bring issues out into the open, it has become acceptable to be overweight or obese.

As promoters of wellness among our employees, it is important to know how to talk transparently about health. You want to be able to ask questions and start conversations. You can start the conversation in a non-confrontational way by saying, "Here are some of the programs that can help you on your journey." By offering educational opportunities, you can start to build a culture of wellness that invites health to the table of conversation among all employees, not only the HR department. In our own organization, we talk about health every day and are very open and honest about it. That has only happened after years of employees becoming more informed.

OUR EXAMPLE

The first speaker we brought in was Brendan Brazier, the author of *Thrive*. He talked about what he does in his own life and about his journey. I remember someone asking him what he ate for breakfast that morning, and his answer was, "I ate two handfuls of cherries and a handful of almonds. That gives me enough energy for my workout, and I feel great." I could see it in the eyes of everyone there. They were thinking: *So we don't have to eat these elaborate meals? If we eat very simply, we can get the nourishment our body needs?* Those types of eye-opening moments are critical for those who attend speaking events like these. For me, that moment showed me just how important education is.

We also brought in Dr. Caldwell Esselstyn from the Cleveland Clinic. I remember him talking about a study he did where there were seventeen to eighteen patients with some level of cardiac disease and clogging of the arteries and veins. He put them all on a high-carb, whole-food, plant-based diet with low fat. He showed scans of their vascular systems. Over several months, the plaque clogging the veins and arteries had disappeared. When he showed the group that it is possible to heal yourself with your diet, everyone was blown away. He also talked about inflammation, which leads to less longevity and chronic disease. He talked about how certain foods are more alkaline, while others are more acidic; the acidic foods cause a lot of inflammation in our bodies, which makes us sick. He explained how most processed foods and animal products are dehydrating, which can lead to more inflammation. His conclusion: the more fruits and vegetables we eat, the more hydrated we will be. The content was highly engaging, especially coming from a doctor at the Cleveland Clinic who had been working in this area for a long time.

Besides inviting speakers, the CHIP program has also been a huge success for our employees. One of our employees was about fifty pounds overweight at fifty years old. She ate a standard American diet and thought she was pretty healthy. She was excited to sign up for CHIP and jumped in with both feet forward. After four or five months, she lost fifty pounds. It was truly amazing. Her cholesterol and her blood pressure went down; all of her labs improved dramatically. Thanks to the education and the support she was getting from CHIP, she was able to make the changes she needed. She started eating a whole-food, plant-based diet and moving more. She even started completing some 5Ks. It is likely she would have never done any of that on her own. Knowing that her company believed in her encouraged her. By taking part in a single educational opportunity offered by her employer, she changed her life.

TRIAL AND ERROR

Trial and error is part of education. For example, some of the speakers we brought in were much more popular than others. Since we are in healthcare, doctors resonated more with our staff because they are seen as experts. If you are going to bring in speakers, look at your mix of employees and try to get speakers who are most applicable to the masses. Early on, we were trying to bring in as many speakers as we could, but we found that a more targeted approach is actually better. It's also important to vary the times speakers come in. We would try to have speakers give two or three different talks, in the morning, evening, and also maybe at lunchtime. If you are going to spend time and money investing in an educational opportunity, you want to make sure it is accessible to your employees.

Some trial and error might be necessary with books and documentaries too. We live in a fast-paced society, and fewer people are reading books. Some employees are not willing to spend eight to ten hours reading a book, but most are willing to pop in a DVD at night and watch a ninety-minute documentary. Have books available for those who prefer reading, but also recognize that documentaries can be extremely powerful. We offered a lot of articles and books in the beginning, but we gained more traction from the documentaries. We would even show a documentary in a theater on the weekends. We offered a showing of *Forks Over Knives* to our employees, and it impacted a lot of people. Other good ones to have available are *What the Health* and *Cowspiracy*. Watching a documentary is a short time commitment, and the images will stick with the viewers.

OTHER EDUCATIONAL INITIATIVES

There are endless tools you can provide your employees for their continued education. Here are a few ideas. First, we provide various brochures in our cafeteria. We also started putting all nutritional information about all of our food in the cafeteria, so everyone could see and understand what choices they were making. We have stations where we talk about different foods. We also have cooking demonstrations in the cafeteria as a way to show employees how to make healthy food at home.

We started a free yoga program; classes are offered early in the morning and right after work. Employees love that, and it's offered at no cost to them. We also built a meditation room, which is a quiet place where employees or physicians can go at any point during the day. In healthcare, in particular, where we are dealing with a high level of stress, intensity, emotions, and sickness, it's important to take a step away from all of that and recharge.

We encourage our employees to attend our city's annual Vegfest, which features speakers and other resources on health and nutrition. Out of these educational opportunities have come things like our jumpstart program, which enables physicians to prescribe food instead of medicine. We offer five to ten days of whole, plant-based food. Sometimes, we charge for the food, and other times it's free. This gives the patient ten days to jump into healthier eating.

As mentioned earlier, a great educational resource is an employee who has already experienced success in a particular area. We link interested employees with these individuals. This one-on-one relationship can be what helps someone make an important change, and leaders in your organization need to be able to identify employees who are willing to be a resource.

After a couple of years, I had a number of employees who had tremendous success. Out of that group, a handful were also great listeners and motivators. They connected easily with other employees and were always willing to help and tell their stories. One woman, whom we'll call Samantha, had lost about fifty pounds and totally changed her life. Not only did she accomplish her goal, but she has always been a remarkable person. When I would refer an employee to her, she would spend hours with that person initially and over the coming months, providing them with resources and answering a significant number of questions about her experience.

Having this kind of mentor and sounding board can be extremely important when making any life or habit changes. These individuals can help others by inviting them to make their goals public and put them out into the universe. Once your goals are public, you are accountable to everyone who knows. Not only that, but now you have support to help you on your bad days.

Again, having a wide range of speakers was also a great idea. For us, that looked like Dr. Greger coming in and talking about the science of nutrition and health. He gave specific scientific information and clinical studies, which resonated with a lot of people. He was very good at giving us the proof that we wanted. Dr. Esselstyn talked about hard-to-digest foods. Eating these foods takes away energy our bodies need to heal, to get rid of toxins, or to perform certain immune functions, which is why we need lighter foods like fruits and vegetables.

WHEN LEARNING CLICKS

I was watching TV with my daughter and wife a while back, and my wife asked me to turn on something about animals. I went to the Animal Planet and turned on *The Crocodile Hunter*. The host was in Africa with giant Nile crocodiles. The crocodiles were eating giant hippos. Several times throughout the hour-long episode, the crocodiles would finish eating, get out of the water, and go lie on the land, not moving for a long period of time. They had giant, distended bellies from all of the hippo meat. They needed to lie still in the sun to digest the food; the sun warmed them, getting their body temperatures up enough to digest the heavy meal. It was then that Dr. Esselstyn's talk finally clicked for me. When I eat a heavy meal and wake up in the middle of the night sweating, it's because my core temperature has risen to help me digest the heavy foods. I'm taking a lot of energy from my body to raise my core temperature and digest these heavy foods. When I eat lighter, simpler foods, my body needs less energy to digest, and more energy can go toward a healthy detox. The simple lesson: don't eat any hippos.

Learning often happens that way. Insight takes a while to fully sink in, but it has to start somewhere. Insight takes full effect when we experience what we have learned in real life. Once employees learn and then have success (weight loss, better sleep, less stress), they'll want to learn even more. They'll be more inspired to seek out opportunities for education and health awareness. They'll be seeking the mind-body-spirit union, to truly take ownership of their health in all areas, not just one. People also tend to want to help others once they find some success themselves.

I remember an employee who came into my office one day and told me about her dinner the night before. She had eaten a lighter meal and felt better. She told me how she slept better and felt great when she woke up. She experienced that simple aha moment when the new insight "clicks." Once that happens for anyone, the sky's the limit because knowledge has turned into experience. For this employee, it was not enough to hear repeated messages about healthy living at work. She had to take action using a trial-and-error approach in order to have the vision to make a lifestyle change for the better.

As you consider what educational opportunities to pursue as part of your wellness program, it's important to remember that food should be the central focus of everything you do. We'll consider why food is so important and how to focus on it in the next chapter.

CHAPTER 5

FOOD IS MEDICINE

Of all the things you can do for your employees, helping them understand and appreciate healthy eating is probably the most important. An improvement in diet leads directly to an improvement in overall health and, more specifically, in chronic disease management. "Food is medicine" comes from Hippocrates, the father of medicine. He said, "Let food be thy medicine, and medicine be thy food." In our organization, we have fully embraced that philosophy, and I would encourage you to do so as well.

MAKING CHANGES HAPPEN

The most basic way to focus on food is by providing healthier options to employees. People want to eat healthier, but doing so is not always convenient or affordable. Healthy food sometimes doesn't taste as good as unhealthy food. If you can provide food that is healthy, affordable, and delicious, your employees will eat healthier.

It is easy for companies to talk about this goal, but it is sometimes difficult to actually make it happen. You might be worried, for example, that employees will be upset if you make changes, especially in an area as personal as food. You will need to have a great deal of confidence in your plan. Know the timelines for the changes you will make, and tell your employees about those changes before they arrive. This gives everyone time to adjust.

When people start seeing the changes in action, they believe the ideas are becoming a reality, and they will be ready for more changes that will come.

OFFERING ALTERNATIVES

The way we helped our employees change their diets in a positive way was by simply providing more fresh foods, more fruits and vegetables, more lower-fat foods, and more options that are vegetarian, vegan, or plant based. One simple change every company can do is to stock the vending machines with healthier snacks, like nuts and healthy bars, rather than candy and soda.

One doctor at our hospital loved to drink some of the new, high-sugar and high-caffeine carbonated beverages. She was not happy when those were eliminated from the vending machines. We had a few tough conversations, but in the end I could at least get her to agree that those beverages have no redeeming health benefits. When these kinds of conversations are necessary, it can be tough to stick with the plan and to not question if these initiatives are hurting rather than helping your organization. The bottom line remains: doing what is best for your team will be best for your company.

Not everyone will be happy with the changes, of course. You need to know when employees might complain. People usually understand when high-sugar items (soda and other carbonated beverages, for example) are eliminated, but you'll get more pushback with a category like dairy. That's when people will say, "Hey, what's going on?" With these categories, you need to be ready to have alternatives. If you make your goals clear and say, "We're going healthy," employees are not going to question the choice of ditching candy and soda. However, many food categories are not as obviously unhealthy. In those cases, it's a good idea to carry the normal items as well as alternatives.

As for expense, do your best to offer each alternative at a similar price as the original. Meat and animal products are expensive. You should be able to offer plant-based foods at a similar price. In some cases, you may even be able to offer healthy alternatives for a lower cost. If you make a plant-based dish of beans and rice or another type of vegetable casserole, for example, you can make a lot of it at once and sell it for a low price.

There are some simple ways to add alternatives rather than eliminate foods altogether. For example, instead of eliminating milk, we changed the milk options. We now only offer skim milk as well as almond, soy, and cashew milk. We did not eliminate cheeseburgers, but we added several alternative burgers, like a black-bean burger and, most recently, something we named the "Impossible" burger. No one can believe it is vegan. People have been willing to try these alternatives and have realized they taste great and cost the same. Once they try the alternative and like it, they'll continue to buy it, and their health will improve. Remember: generally speaking, most people want to eat healthier. If you make a healthy diet convenient, affordable, and tasty, they'll make the healthier choice.

GRADUAL SHIFT

As with other parts of the process, don't try to overhaul your approach to food all at once. This goes back to having a plan and setting the expectation; you should plan to make changes over several years, not all in one month. One month, make one change, and the next month, make another. Some months, you might make bigger changes, like eliminating soda; other months, you might make smaller changes, like adding almond milk in the cafeteria. The key is to be intentional about heading down the path of wellness. Allow employees to come along with you on the journey, rather than making them angry with changes they are not prepared to handle.

A big piece of the puzzle is to get employees to try new things, little by little. Many of us think we eat a variety of foods, but in truth, we don't. We eat the same things every week, or even every day. Some of us always have cereal for breakfast, for example, or bacon and eggs. At lunch, we always have a sandwich or a salad. Dinner is always either chicken, burgers, or pizza. Most people eat what they like and repeat that pattern. Having alternatives added gradually at work helps them branch out, little by little, and start making different, healthier choices.

Gradual change is important, not just for the wellness plan to succeed, but for your overall culture. If you move fast and eliminate certain items without any lead time or communication, employees will feel as if the company is imposing its will on them. They may feel the company doesn't value them or care about them as individuals. When you do decide to eliminate something (soda, for example), give a significant amount of lead time and communicate about it. Even offer some education around the choice. If it's part of the plan and everyone knows it is coming, they will be more willing to accept the change. Ultimately, you win by keeping your employees engaged and feeling valued.

OUR EXAMPLE

As we made gradual changes over time, we decided on the primary foods we wanted to change. One was butter. We removed all butter from the hospital and now offer alternatives like Earth Balance. We still get some push-back, which is interesting because butter is an oil and fat. There's no nutritional value, and I don't think people know that. They just like the taste. Of course, employees who simply cannot go without butter can bring it from home.

We also decided to make a clear change with milk. We still have milk in the hospital cafeteria, but only skim milk, which is healthier than 2 percent or whole milk. We are especially promoting the milk alternatives. In making the milk switch, we learned the importance of display. We crowd out the less healthy options to display the alternative front and center. People get excited about the options. They've said, "I can have almond, soy, or cashew milk! This is fantastic." No one says, "Give me less options." This is America; we love options.

Another major change we made, which came later down

the road, was with fried foods. We eliminated fried food in our cafeteria and physically got rid of the fryers. You'd be hard-pressed to find anyone who would say fried food is healthy. Employees couldn't honestly make a case for it. By baking instead of frying, we haven't changed the types of food being offered, but the way it's prepared. We didn't get much pushback in this area. In fact, a lot of employees have actually enjoyed how baked food tastes.

We also decided to offer more vegan and vegetarian options. Daily, we now have nonmeat and nonanimal product options. Our team experiments with different recipes, sees what sells and what doesn't, and asks for feedback. The vegan and vegetarian meals are often much more flavorful than meat, which is not that flavorful without ketchup or steak sauce. When you eat living foods—vegetables and grains, for example—they are naturally more flavorful.

The good news is that no one will give pushback about expanding the salad bar. A lot of people like to eat salads for lunch, and a bigger salad bar means more options. Of course, you want to offer alternatives to cheese and unhealthy salad dressings. When people layer those on their salads, they end up becoming unhealthy.

DISPLAY KITCHEN

We are in the process of creating an actual display kitchen, which is similar to a cooking class. A chef, teacher, or coach creates a recipe in front of people, showing them how to cook certain foods in a healthy way. People enjoy watching so they can learn how food is prepared. When we learn to cook, we know how the food is prepared, which is important to living a healthy lifestyle.

In our cafeteria already, we have a display cooking area where we are cooking in front of employees. We haven't offered classes yet, but employees do get to see our chefs creating salads, wraps, and more. We have several stations where we create food in front of our employees. They love seeing all the ingredients that go into their food and how it's prepared. This focus on displaying food preparation helps people eat healthier. For us, it has increased interest among employees, and more are willing to try new foods when they see them being made. When they then find out that the food actually tastes good, they'll likely come back for more.

Our plan for the display kitchen is ultimately to offer classes before or after work, not during the workday. Some cities have display kitchens that companies could use. In that case, the company could pay for employees to go take a class or could offer an incentive for a date night at a class. These classes motivate employees to cook at home, which is healthier than eating out. Unfortunately, it's a lost art. There will also be less sodium or added oils and sugars in your meals cooked at home. The more you can offer your employees opportunities to learn how to cook at home, the healthier they will be.

If you're going to encourage employees to cook at home, you also have to encourage work-life balance. Help them carve out time in their lives to cook. Encourage them that the time they give each day to preparing their food is worth it. To make the task of preparation easier, you might suggest meal-delivery companies like Purple Carrot, which offer plant-based alternatives. They ship you all of the ingredients and the recipe for a meal, and then you prepare it. It makes healthy food prep really simple.

PARTNERSHIPS

Another way we have encouraged employees to eat healthier is by offering them discounts to local healthy restaurants. A discount may not be enough to get them to change their eating habits, but it may make an employee a little more likely to at least give it a try. See if you can work out a partnership with a local restaurant to offer discounts to your employees. Many restaurants will be open to this because it gets people in their door. In our hospital, where we provide the healthy food, we do provide a discount to our employees, physicians, and volunteers. From a price perspective, we are one of the least expensive "restaurants" in town. We are lucky we have a captive audience.

FINANCIAL CONSIDERATIONS

Many companies think that offering vegetarian and vegan food will be more expensive, but that is not the case. If you look at your grocery receipt, you will see that meat and animal products are the expensive items, while simple foods like rice, beans, and quinoa are not—not to mention that you can buy these in bulk. Fruit and vegetables will be more expensive, but you can charge a little more for these. Employees understand fruits and vegetables are a little more expensive. That said, don't charge $3 for an apple. You can charge $1 or $0.75 for an apple, and people will see that as a fair price. Price transparency is key.

Eating healthy is not necessarily going to be more expensive for your employees either, but if they can get a meal that is fresh, tastes great, and is convenient, they will probably be willing to pay a little more. They will consider that it is worth it to feel better and not have the food coma after lunch. All of a sudden, they will notice their body isn't using so much energy on digestion, and they have more energy to work.

We didn't think our sales would go up in our cafeteria when we started offering healthier options, but they did. Many of our employees liked the tasty, healthy alternatives and stopped bringing in their own lunches as often. The convenience factor was huge. When you work all day and have kids at home, the last thing you want to do is make yourself a lunch for work the next day, after you have already made dinner and the kids' lunches for the next day. If you could save twenty minutes a night and know you are going to get a great meal at a fair price, then that will become your choice more often than not. We saw sales continue to grow because people enjoyed what we were offering.

Even if you do not have a cafeteria, there is likely still a lot of food around your office—perhaps a lot of unhealthy food like cookies and donuts. One simple and low-cost option is to have whole fruit delivered to the office every week for employees. At the least, your employees now have an option. If all that's in the break room is donuts, everyone will grab one. If there is also fresh fruit, employees have to make a choice. More often than you might think, people will make the healthy choice.

THE IMPACT OF FOOD

Food has been central to my own health journey over the years. If I had to choose one area to focus on in my own life or had to encourage an employee to focus on only one area, it would be right here. How we eat impacts our lives in every way.

Simple changes can make a big difference. For example, one change I made in my diet was to eat less fat. Fat is important to our bodies, but how much do we really need? Food that is high in fat usually has a higher concentration of calories and can help stave off hunger for a few hours when we can't eat a meal. However, I found that eating fat at every meal left me feeling heavy. When I started eating more fruits and whole grains, my body felt it was getting a constant stream of nutrition. It was no longer experiencing the peaks and valleys that come from a diet heavy in fat. With that simple change, I slept better and was able to lose those last five pounds that had always been the toughest to lose to get to my ideal body weight.

Food should be our medicine and not our vice. It should refuel us and heal us, not make us feel exhausted and sick. In our own company, I have seen the way people's lives have changed when they changed the way they ate. This is why I place such a large emphasis on food in any wellness program.

It is, indeed, the most important part of a wellness program. Yet it can be the most difficult piece to implement. I want to encourage you to stick with it. Keep advocating for positive change, little by little. Keep educating people in your company that a poor diet causes chronic disease, puts people in the hospital, and causes health insurance costs to skyrocket. If, as a company, you can change the food employees put in their bodies, you can bend the cost curve for keeping your employees healthy. Sometimes, employees need incentives to begin down the road to healthier eating and a healthier lifestyle. We will discuss how incentives can drive change in the next chapter.

CHAPTER 6

CREATING A SUSTAINABLE CULTURE OF HEALTHY LIVING

When people start getting healthier, they get excited. They have more energy and then want to tell others about their success. Healthy food is the gateway to this state of more awareness. It allows a person to live more in the moment, which leads to a greater interest in the environment and even spirituality. The excitement that comes with health is pervasive; it spreads throughout an organization, which is crucial for momentum.

As the leader of an organization, it is your job to recognize the people who are having success and then recruit them to spread their message to others. This begins a grassroots effort by ambassadors who have had success, promoting wellness. The wellness movement at this point can often become self-sustaining. Your job as the leader is to help amplify these stories; give other leaders and employees a podium, whether literally or metaphorically, to tell their stories.

CELEBRATING SUCCESSES THROUGH SHARING STORIES

In our organization, we have heard many amazing stories over the years. We do our best to spotlight these in any way we can. I will share just a few.

As employees get healthier, some get very involved in athletics. Over the last couple of years, several of our employees have completed their first triathlon. I remember when a couple of them came up to me and said, "We're going to do an Ironman." An Ironman is a long race! It's a 2.4-mile swim, a 112-mile bike ride, and a 26.2-mile run. These are employees who had not been athletes. The wellness movement we started inspired them enough to take action. They had more energy because they were eating better, so they started running, swimming, and biking. After a year and a half, they were doing the Ironman triathlon. Anything is possible.

One employee, Ronald, who was previously semi-obese and had never worked out much or lived a healthy lifestyle, came up to me recently and said, "Josh, I'm doing my first triathlon and need your help." He'd lost a lot of weight and had been swimming, biking, and running. People like him are very inspiring. His goal now is to beat me in this triathlon, and I think he can. His confidence in his ability to shape and move his body in a way he never thought he could is just amazing. He feels empowered, and he credits our organization for offering educational opportunities and painting a picture of what he could achieve. He now has a great story to share with other employees. I tell his story to others and connect him with others whenever I get the chance.

Another employee, Steve, had stage-four cancer and was told he had ninety to 120 days to live. He was not ready to die, so he did some research and began an "extreme diet." He ate only living, whole foods. He drank a lot of raw vegetable juice and smoothies and ate raw foods, especially fruits and vegetables. He totally detoxed his body. A year and a half later, he was cancer free. Everyone was amazed. I know his story has inspired many other employees to make changes.

One of my supervisors, Rose, was close to retirement when she began having headaches. She found out she had a brain tumor behind her eye. It was about the size of a quarter, but because it was behind her eye, it was inoperable. Surgeons couldn't remove it without damaging her brain or killing her. She was given three months to live. The news was, of course, devastating to her and to her family. I gave her a couple of books: *The China Study* by T. Colin Campbell and *Thrive* by Brendan Brazier. I wanted her to feel empowered to know there were still things she could do. I referred her to the employee mentioned above, who had beaten stage-four cancer, and they talked over a series of months. She became educated about food and health and how to detox her body, and as a result, her tumor shrunk until it eventually went away. She worked for us for another three years and then retired. Currently, she is still leading a healthy life.

People with cancer are facing many unknowns, but one thing they can control is what they put into their bodies. Many employees heard these stories and were inspired by the idea that a healthy lifestyle can play a major role in curing chronic disease. I have seen employees use diet to reverse cardiovascular disease, autoimmune disease, and rheumatoid arthritis as well. When they decided to change what they were eating, their bodies were able to remove the toxins, healing naturally. When you cut your finger, it heals on its own. Your body can heal small injuries and chronic diseases, too, if you give it the fuel it needs to heal. Sure, it takes more time and energy to heal from cancer or cardiac disease, but if you put your body into a balanced pH state, the immune system will be able to fight off disease. Put hydrating, alkalizing foods into your body, and the body can heal itself. These stories are proof.

Once you start hearing these kinds of stories come to the surface, the next step is to figure out how to have these employees share their stories. Nine times out of ten, they will at least be willing to mentor other employees on an individual basis, even if they don't want to get up on a stage and share publicly. If they are willing to share in front of a group, take advantage of this and set aside some time to have them do just that.

RECOGNITION

When it comes to recognizing employees for their successes, check with them first on how they would like to be recognized. Some would like to be recognized monetarily; others simply appreciate a "good job." Some would like to see their name in the newspaper; others would like to receive an award in front of lots of people and then give a speech. Be sure to ask them what they would prefer.

Also, be sure to keep checking in with employees about their goals. If an employee's goal is to lose weight, help him remember that it's a journey. They didn't put on the weight overnight or even over a month. It goes on slowly, and it comes off slowly. Keep checking in with them, recognizing them in small ways when you can. Almost everyone who loses weight is encouraged by being recognized publicly because it's hard to do and it's exciting. It feels fantastic when someone says, "Hey, it looks like you've lost weight." Even if they haven't, this type of comment gives people the stamina to keep going. Then, when they start seeing the benefits—more energy, better sleep, lower stress, increased productivity, more desire to exercise—they will continue down that path because they will want to achieve the next level.

As a company, you might consider including a health and wellness goal in annual evaluations. You can have a company-wide goal to lose two thousand pounds, for example. You can also have individual health goals that get discussed at an employee's annual review. Perhaps employees who meet a goal can receive a bonus. The bonus provides incentive for them to stick with it.

MAKING STORIES PERSONAL

Once you have employees on the front lines who have experienced success, others get excited. "If they did it, I can do it too" becomes a common mantra. Other employees will work toward having their own story. They will seek out resources and education, and become very intentional about seeing changes, not because their company or their friend told them to do it, but because they now want to do it. That is key.

Moreover, they now know who they can reach out to if they need guidance or advice along the way. One reason why it's important to promote current success stories of employees is because most employees don't want to go to their boss and say, "How did you achieve results?" They want to go to the person in the cubicle next to them; it's a much more personal and comfortable conversation.

TANGIBLE INCENTIVES

Incentives are a great way to recognize employees who go above and beyond. We have a pool of money we use to give cash awards to employees who are very deserving. We might give an award to an employee who is going above and beyond or doing exceptional work in their jobs, but we also might give one to an individual working hard on improving their health. The Ironman triathletes each received an award, for example. We recognized how inspirational their efforts were.

We have not yet tried cash incentives tied to certain smaller health goals, but we have asked, "What if?" A lot of organizations are already doing these types of incentives, especially health insurance companies. As we look ahead, we are considering incentives for employees who reach certain metrics. If, for example, employees are encouraged to hit a target weight by the end of the year for a $1,000 or $2,000 bonus, most would hit that weight.

That's a lot of money! Yet, from the company's perspective, giving $1,000 or $2,000 to an employee who reached their weight-loss goal is much cheaper than paying up to $30,000 for a hospital stay. Bonuses are a smart idea; they are the future. Consider giving bonuses for any health metric, including blood pressure, cholesterol, or labs.

Insurance companies have really led the way in this space. Many plans now offer cash bonuses to entice their members to stay healthy. They might pay $50 for getting your annual wellness visit and $25 for going to the gym ten times or logging over five hundred minutes of physical activity. I have seen rewards for completing a 5K or for getting a flu shot. It makes sense. Insurance companies want to keep their members out of the hospital as well. In the end, it saves the company a lot of money.

The incentive doesn't have to be cash related, though. We have also given prizes like Fitbits, which allow people to track their steps and their heart rate. We've given massages, pedicures/manicures, and spa days. We are also planning to give away healthy trips, whether it's a retreat or a spa for the weekend, or a cruise for connecting mind, body, and spirit. These types of incentives make the wellness journey very exciting and work well for employees who are at higher risk, in terms of their health. Incentives make it clear the company is invested in its employees' success. Again, the cost of the incentives is nothing compared to the cost of sick employees with hospital stays. Paying for incentives up front is more cost-effective than paying for healthcare and insurance costs later on.

Personal goals can also become incentives for some individuals. Deciding to run a marathon is a big goal. If a person is training for a marathon, in general she will be a healthier person because she is moving her body more and burning calories. Setting the goal, in and of itself, becomes an incentive for employees to stay active.

BIOMARKERS

Though there are privacy rules, most companies have general health data on their employees. Insurance companies do too. They put employees into pools of high, moderate, and low risk for hospitalization or other health events. Once you have baseline data, you can create individualized goals. Those could include a certain amount of weight that is lost by a certain date, blood pressure down to a certain level by a certain date, or cholesterol at a certain reading by a certain date. The goal could be to get off medications altogether or reduce the number of medications that are being taken daily. Since prescriptions are a high cost to any company, the more prescriptions you can eliminate, the better for everyone.

HEALTHY CAMARADERIE

Healthy camaraderie means everyone is in this fight together. We are all on the journey to health. Sharing stories and offering incentives provides excitement, but ultimately, employees want to know they are part of a team. They want to know that they can interact with their team members about what they're doing for their health. Weight loss and healthy eating are much more difficult when they are not public goals. Without camaraderie, it's too easy to have the cookies and ice cream at night and tell yourself you'll do better tomorrow. When you have a team holding you accountable, you don't want to let the team down.

We have seen the effect of this kind of camaraderie, even on a county level. Our county put together something called the Million Mile Movement. Everyone involved logged their miles—walking, running, or biking. As a county, we were trying to get to one million miles. The effort created buy-in from a lot of people, and it built lots of excitement around health.

COMPANY CULTURE

The end goal of wellness programs and movements is to have a highly productive company with a thriving corporate culture. You want an environment where employees are engaged and excited to be there. They work well with their colleagues, and there is a sense of teamwork.

A wellness movement is a vehicle to create part of that culture because it does bring people together. It inspires conversations about health, wellness, food, spirituality, and more. People find they have a lot in common with their coworkers, and they start spending time together outside of work. It's a self-sustaining kind of culture, and it's one companies should want. Your employees will pay you back tenfold over the investment you give them.

Culture is often defined as the "way we do it here." This definition became a reality for us when the team started believing we really cared for them and their health. They became invested in the company. They went from being "renters" to "owners." The shift in our culture was made clear by conversations I would have with our customers (our patients and families). They could not stop gushing about the warm atmosphere, the teamwork, the smiles, and the personal connections they had with the team. The employees went above and beyond and were able to solve issues that were sometimes outside of their scope of responsibility because they felt empowered to be owners and problem solvers. Stories about staff coming to see patients on their time off, or throwing birthday celebrations for patients, were common. Our employee engagement scores soared, which positively impacted results all around, including our patient experience scores and our bottom-line financials.

Creating a sense of teamwork can go beyond the four

walls and out into the community. We will take some time to consider what a wellness community looks like in the next chapter.

CHAPTER 7

WELLNESS COMMUNITY

In the United States right now, there is a significant movement around health and food. By and large, we are a sick, obese nation, and people are getting tired of it. They're asking questions and reconsidering what they think they know about healthy living. These conversations happening throughout each community are connecting people. There's a true sense that others are on the same page.

These same conversations are happening in the workplace community as well. Health, weight management, and other topics that were once hidden are now in the light; people are much more transparent. There's no longer a stigma attached to talking about health and disease. Take the elderly, for example. They'll tell you every ailment they have and what medication they're taking. In general, conversations around health have become much more open. This is good news for your wellness program, and it allows you the opportunity to connect more broadly with the community.

COMMUNITY OF DOCTORS

With more focus and more conversations around health and wellness, doctors are focused on treating the whole person, not just one symptom. Doctors are no longer interested in simply writing a prescription and sending patients on their way. They want to figure out exactly what's wrong with patients, and they're spending more time with their patients to really listen to them and connect the dots.

Companies have an opportunity to let their employees know about the doctors who are treating the whole person. Word of mouth helps to know which doctors might be a good fit. As with food, this is about offering alternative choices, not taking anything away. Before making any healthcare decision, employees should seek to get educated and understand issues and options available to them. Access to more opinions and more options is always better.

In our community, we noticed certain doctors were achieving great results with patients, and we wanted our employees to achieve these results as well. We used word of mouth to let employees know about these opportunities. These doctors were spending more time with patients, providing more information, and discussing nutrition. They were prescribing whole-food jumpstart programs—food for ten days if the patient would try a whole-food, plant-based diet. This is where new food pharmacies come in. Instead of a doctor prescribing a pill, they'll prescribe food. The patient will go to the food pharmacy to fill their prescription for healthy, living foods.

WE ARE ALL CONNECTED

Recently, a local firefighter in our community had a stroke and came into the hospital. He was in his early forties and had two young children at home. He looked like he was in great shape, so it was surprising he had a stroke. Fortunately for him, we have an amazing team of physicians and employees at the hospital who are trained in the care of complex strokes and who save lives every day. We treated him, and he regained full use of his body and his mind. Afterward, though, he asked himself, "Why did I have a stroke? I'm healthy. I work out. I'm in great shape." That's when he took time to learn about nutrition. He started eating a whole-food, plant-based diet and got healthier and healthier. I tell this story to illustrate how everyone is in this together. If people in our community who are firefighters, police officers, healthcare workers, and neighbors are not talking about health, the lack of communication can be devastating to a community. Luckily, this firefighter recovered, but not everyone is that lucky. The community—the families, the neighbors—is affected every time it loses someone.

In each community, we need to continue to help each other. As a company, we can help by providing education to our employees. If you are a company with a large footprint, the work you do within your company will spill out over into your community. Employees who have achieved results in your organization should promote health and wellness not only within the company but also within the community. The more they can create a movement on a community level, the better off everyone will be. The movement will encourage citizens to vote with their credit cards at the grocery stores by buying healthier foods. It will encourage citizens to talk to their local leaders about health and wellness, even about the food that goes into school lunches.

More and more people are joining the movement and getting excited about it. People are trying to understand health and wellness and are trying to take better care of their bodies. They are thinking about what they are putting into their bodies and thinking about moving their bodies. More healthy businesses are opening. More people walk or ride their bike, instead of driving or taking the bus.

People are making health a priority. It's a movement our community has embraced. Naturally, as a hospital and healthcare system, we view ourselves as the community resource for health and wellness. When you come to one of our hospitals, we want you to understand that health and healing are our number-one priority. I believe, however, that every community can embrace this same mission.

If you live in a smaller community where there isn't local access to certain information, speakers, or healthy food, get online. The internet has made information accessible to everyone. You can find a physician, nutrition plans, diet plans, and workout plans. Google "how to train for an Ironman." Where you live is no longer a limiting factor. If there's a will, there's a way. If you want to be intentional about your health and wellness, the resources are out there. You only have to seek them out.

Another way to take your wellness program to the next level, besides community involvement, is by beginning to use data. Data gathering can provide large returns for your company. The next chapter will show you why.

CHAPTER 8

DATA GATHERING AND USE

As organizations start to look at taking their wellness programs to the next level, data becomes important. Understanding what employees are facing, what they are at risk for, and who the high-risk employees are is key. Once you know this information, you can focus on trying to intervene with resources to get employees moving in the right direction.

Keep in mind: data gathering and analysis are next-level tasks to be done once your wellness program is well underway and thriving. It is for this reason that this is the final chapter of the book. That said, data can be highly valuable to your company. It can help you clarify your target audience for your wellness initiative and identify the high-risk employees.

In a typical company, all employees pay a similar rate for health insurance depending on their plan. There is little differentiation based on risk. If an individual shops for health insurance in the marketplace, though, that's different. Insurance companies stratify individuals by risk, and the ones at highest risk pay more. In a company, that's not the case. With a company, an insurance company identifies the number of people who need to be insured and how many of those people are at high risk and then gives a flat rate for the entire company. The higher the number of high-risk employees, the higher the flat rate will be, which everyone usually shares equally.

Wouldn't it be better if health data were used to more fairly charge employees? Obviously, this would be a better scenario for the lower-risk employees who are taking care of their body and health every day. Those who are high-risk would pay higher premiums, while those who are low-risk would pay less. This alone should motivate employees to take better care of themselves, since they would want to be in the lower-cost bracket. This approach would be no different than other types of insurance. With car insurance, you pay more if you have a history of accidents or speeding tickets. With life insurance, you pay more if you have health factors that make you high-risk. Why is it different with health insurance for employees and companies? Data can help.

GATHERING DATA

First and foremost, gathering the data is the most important step, and there are a number of ways to achieve it. Some organizations offer incentives, in the form of cash or gift cards, for employees to get a health screening. These involve blood draws, health questionnaires, and some other testing. This is an effective way not only to get employees to see a doctor but also to get data for your company. The data should provide insight into who is high-risk. Risk is anything from age, weight, and habits (smoking, drinking, etc.) to prior history of medical issues (heart attack, stroke, etc.).

Insurance companies have a large amount of history on their patients, but it's not always easy to access that information. Due to HIPPA privacy laws, you can't access the information an insurance company has on your employees. Employees can grant a company access to their personal history. They can sign off, giving the company rights to see their information as patients to help the company understand the risk profiles of their employees and to provide better education.

Companies should shop around for insurance providers, like they would shop in any other marketplace. They should ask what tools insurance companies have to help them create a healthier population. Insurance companies are motivated, too, to insure healthy people; they don't want expensive claims either. Ask the insurance provider, "What data can you share, and how can we identify employees who are at high risk and get them the education and help they need to become healthier?" You should seek a true partnership. Insurance companies possess important information on employees, and it is important that they can pass that knowledge on to your company.

FINE-TUNING

Once you have the data and know whose risk is higher, you can cater certain testing or educational opportunities to the high-risk population. As you start fine-tuning your wellness initiatives, you will notice the 80-20 rule at work: 20 percent of your employees account for 80 percent of your healthcare costs. The cost could be even higher. In some cases, 10 percent of your employees account for 90 percent of your healthcare costs. It's easy to see why you would want to understand who those people are who make up the 10 percent. While you may not be able to offer every initiative to your entire company because of cost, you will want to offer it to those employees who really need it. You will want to provide them all the help you can—to employ all the strategies we have talked about in this book to support their journey toward wellness.

Various screenings can also help you with fine-tuning.

Anyone over age fifty, for example, should get a colonoscopy. Women over forty should get a mammogram. Data from these screenings will give you more up-to-date data and help employees catch issues early on. If you can't get this data from your insurance company, work with your employees to get it from them. Have them sign the HIPAA release. Explain it's for their good and the good of the whole company. If everyone gets healthier, everyone's insurance rates will come down.

In our organization, we gave gift cards for use toward healthy purchases for everyone who got a full blood profile, and the results were analyzed to determine who was at risk for certain ailments. We used said data to get those higher-risk people the opportunity to participate in some of the initiatives mentioned previously. With our simple incentive, a very high percentage of our employees completed the blood profile. We also invited spouses to take the wellness screening if they were on the company insurance. If spouses are unhealthy, you'll want to know that too. Employees have been on board with this initiative because we explain what we are doing and make it as convenient as possible. The whole process takes thirty to forty minutes.

HEALTHCARE COSTS RELATED TO DATA

In your organization, you will want to find the 20 percent

or 10 percent—those who are regularly in and out of the hospital or on a lot of prescription medications. The needs of this population significantly run up your healthcare bill. Your task is to identify these people and then understand them and how they live. Without understanding, you can't get them the tools and resources they need to help them lead a healthier life. The goal is to help them stop the revolving door of going in to the emergency room or the hospital every month.

Once these employees understand the company cares about them and wants to invest in them and their health, they'll be more willing to try some of the wellness initiatives. Then, they will start to feel better and take more ownership of their health. Until you convince them that you care and want to help, it can be difficult for them to break the cycles on their own. Furthermore, if you don't know who's living the cycle in the first place, it's difficult for you to help them in any direct way.

Often, employees don't even realize the cost of their healthcare to the company. When you have a third-party payer system (the insurance company is paying the hospital bills directly), employees don't necessarily even see the bill. They don't understand how they are driving up healthcare costs for the insurance company, for their company, for their coworkers, and ultimately for themselves. Data helps employees see how they're contributing to the cost of healthcare.

The idea that high-risk employees in companies would pay more for health insurance is still a controversial subject, but I think it will happen in the near future. Companies will not continue to bear the brunt of rising insurance and healthcare costs because of a handful of unhealthy employees who continue to be unhealthy year after year. Eventually, they will pass this cost on to the employees. It's just a matter of time before they decide to make this change.

OUR FINDINGS

Data gathering and use has been extremely successful in our organization. In general, you probably know who is at higher risk just by walking around the company and looking at your employees. If they look tired, stressed, or overweight, they're probably at higher risk. The data just confirms this.

Due to the collection of data, we were able to provide preventative education for countless employees who were in the early stages of chronic disease, including diabetes and coronary heart disease. Due to the mandatory testing, a significant number of team members were able to diagnose their cancer at stage one, giving them a very good chance to cure themselves.

One employee, named Jeff, had blood work done that

indicated possible heart disease. He promptly scheduled himself with a cardiologist and had a diagnostic cardiac catheterization procedure completed. He learned that 80–90 percent of his left coronary artery was blocked with plaque. If he had not known this information, he could have had a heart attack and died suddenly in a matter of weeks. Today, he thanks the company and his leaders for being proactive and helping him stay healthy. To people like Jeff, who have had a close call with death, every day is a blessing.

The data also helped us shift our mindset. It helped us understand that everyone is different; some people take good care of themselves, but others don't know how. It showed us that we needed to provide easy-entry opportunities for the latter group.

Through the screenings we have done, some employees caught their cancer in its early stages, which allowed them to treat it at stage one instead of stage four. We did the screenings two years in a row and collected a large amount of data to utilize. It's a good idea to repeat the screening every few years, since you will most likely add new employees. Repeating it will also help you track if your employees are getting healthier.

One of the most interesting aspects about data gathering is that just about everyone thinks they are healthy. It's not until they have a heart attack or a stroke that they wake up and realize they're not as healthy as they thought. Once our employees were able to see the data we provided them, many became more proactive with preventative activities.

PRODUCTIVITY

The 5-10 percent of your employees who are at higher risk are likely less productive because they don't feel good. We noticed that a good number of our employees in this group had a lot of health-risk factors, which kept them from being super productive at work or elsewhere. It makes sense that they would be less productive if they were not eating right, getting enough sleep, and stressed. The data helped us identify these people so we could do some interventions. As their health improved, their productivity increased.

DATA USE

The data is crucial to helping us all know what to do. Some of us forget that we have control over our health; we tend to think of health as a random force that happens to us. If you have a heart attack or a stroke, you're "unlucky." Science, however, now tells us this is not the case. If you lead an unhealthy lifestyle, you're going to be at a much higher risk for scary health events. Insurance companies have known this for years. They look at an employee and say,

"This person has all these risk factors. They'll probably have a heart attack in the next two years." These events are not random, and we all have a risk profile.

Companies need to understand that with data they have the knowledge and the power to save their employees' lives, not just cut healthcare costs significantly. Companies can intervene and provide opportunities for their employees to take ownership of their health and truly improve it. Insurance companies are less motivated than your company. If healthcare costs for your company go up, they can always raise your rates.

Like I said earlier, companies aren't going to continue to bear the brunt of the cost of healthcare. They will start passing this cost on to employees, especially the higher-risk employees. It behooves employees to take ownership of their health now. We see variable costs with some insurance plans already. If you're a smoker, for example, you'll pay a higher premium. Other health questions aren't yet being asked, but they will be soon enough.

Companies that have the data have an advantage. Yes, some people are genetically inclined to have a heart attack or a stroke. Nonetheless, environmental factors play a larger role in chronic disease. If you understand a person's risk, you can know how to provide intervention. Once you invest in your employees and they get healthier, they will be very committed and loyal to the organization.

CARING FOR THE EMPLOYEE

Since private companies traditionally haven't gotten into the details of people's lives, the conversation around data gathering can be seen as scary. The Affordable Care Act and the open marketplace for health insurance have set the stage for people with higher risk factors paying more for health insurance. Even now, you could be paying $500 a month, while your neighbor is paying $200 a month. You don't know that, though, because it isn't something people talk about. After all, the conversation will be much easier when you have opportunities in place to offer to your employees. Being honest with employees and setting expectations is important too. If you tell an employee she is high-risk, and that the company is looking at changing insurance in a few years to a plan that would charge high-risk employees more, she will hopefully take you up on your offer to help her become healthier. That sets the expectation and gives her time to get into a healthier category.

As leaders, we have to start caring more about our employees as people rather than as workers who punch a time card. We need to continue to move in the direction of caring about the total person. One way we can do this is by being honest with employees about their real status when it comes to health and then supporting them as they get healthier. If we care for our employees, they will become healthier. When they become healthier, healthcare costs will decrease across the board.

CONVERSATION WITH HIGH-RISK EMPLOYEES

Most likely, your employees have never had a boss or a leader want to have a conversation with them about their health. Typically, health is a subject that is not discussed until someone has health issues or is diagnosed with a disease. Unfortunately, it is something we take for granted until we lose it. Below are a few tips for how to start conversations with your employees about their health.

First, do your best to keep these discussions positive. Ask a few questions. What have they done already to improve their health? What are their health goals? Can they write down their goals? Can they share them with you? You never want to come from a place of judgment. You do not know what has happened in this person's life or how they arrived where they are today. You have to go in understanding that you are delving into a personal space. Be encouraging, and discuss where they are and where they want to be in terms of their goals.

The vast majority of the time, people know what they need

to do to be healthy, but that doesn't mean it is easy. That is why it is important to offer practical solutions during your conversation. If you offer education and support, an employee will be much more willing to dive in.

I recommend that during your evaluations with all employees, you build in a time to discuss one or two of their personal health goals. All of us are more motivated by personal goals than goals given to us. If you are open, willing to listen, and show that you truly care in your conversations, your employees will feel part of a family and take action in becoming healthier.

CONCLUSION

THE FUTURE

In the United States, we have the greatest healthcare system in the world. We have amazing doctors who save lives daily. Yet our system is allowing people to sustain unhealthy lifestyles. If you are eating poorly, you end up needing surgery or medication. Healthcare accounts for 17 percent of the US gross domestic product now. People overutilize the system, and that's an understatement. The system is not sustainable. The government currently insures about 130 million people through Medicare, Medicaid, the VA, CHIP, and the Affordable Care Act. In ten years, that number will be about 170 million.[1]

---

1   Centers for Medicare and Medicaid Services, "NHE Fact Sheet," CMS.gov, accessed March 3, 2018, https://www.cms.gov/research-statistics-data-and-systems/statistics-trends-and-reports/nationalhealthexpenddata/nhe-fact-sheet.html.

As healthcare costs continue to rise, we will see more of the cost pushed to individuals—a positive because it makes the cost of healthcare more transparent. There is a moral hazard when a third-party payer like an insurance company pays the bill before a patient ever sees the total cost of their visit. Thankfully, greater transparency is on the horizon. Before long, purchasing healthcare will be more like buying groceries; you will know the cost of everything when you place it in your shopping cart.

GOOD NEWS

The good news is that we can expect a happier, healthier future. Even more important than changes in healthcare, the health and wellness movement, with a focus on prevention, is gaining traction nationally. People are trying to educate themselves; there is endless information on the internet and lots of books and documentaries too. People are sick of being sick; they're seeing that the elderly are not thriving in their golden years, and that's scary. They're tired of not having access to good food. They're tired of going to the hospital. So they're taking charge, and that's exciting.

There is a lot of data available now too. We have much more understanding on the state of people's health. This is especially true for the younger generations, which are growing up with information at their fingertips. They are seeing the baby boomers suffer with chronic diseases, and they are saying, "I don't want that to be me." They are getting educated and doing all they can to learn how they can prevent illness and lead healthier lifestyles.

There is hope. Information is getting out there, and there are countless success stories. Some of the best documentaries, such as *Forks Over Knives*, *Cowspiracy*, and *What the Health*, to name a few, are helping people learn about their health and inspiring them to get off the conveyor belt of chronic disease. Documentaries hold an enormous amount of power because of the visuals, and our culture connects with them on a deep level.

People in this movement are taking notice of celebrities dying young. It's in the news every week. We don't expect celebrities to die at fifty-five. Just fifty years ago, cancer was not as widespread as it is today. It wasn't even talked about very much. If you knew someone who had cancer, you were in the minority, but today, everyone knows someone who has been affected by cancer. All of this has encouraged many more people to take ownership of their health.

THE RIPPLE EFFECT

Remember: it starts with you. You have to be the first to take ownership of your own health. First, get the knowledge you need and change your own life. Once you do that, you can help others. People will seek you out because you will be a lighthouse.

Remember: healthy living is a journey, not a destination. No one has yet figured out how to live to 130. If you ask ten different centenarians how they lived to one hundred, you'll get ten different answers. We think we know, but then we realize that maybe we don't know. This journey takes a village. It takes a community to continue to get educated and help each other. Whether at the organization or community level, we all can help one another, as we all still have a lot to learn.

Remember: the goal is to create a culture of wellness. A wellness program is just one way to do that. The mission is to help people lead healthier lives, and this program is a great way to support that mission.

BACK TO MY STORY

For me, getting healthy was the best thing I've ever done. Until you get healthy, you don't realize how much of a fog you have lived in. Once you start to eat healthier, you lose that fog, and your energy and mental clarity go way up. You start to live more in the moment. Your interactions become deeper and your relationships more meaningful. Getting healthy helped me figure out what's important in life, so that I could focus on living, not just going from one day to the next on the hamster wheel.

When I made a personal decision to fully pursue a healthy life, people noticed the change in me. They noticed my energy level had gone up. They looked at me and knew something was different. They would often say, "Hey, you look really good," but they couldn't put their finger on it. They didn't know why I looked better. A combination of a better diet, better sleep, and better stress management had done the trick.

When you're in the cycle of living an unhealthy lifestyle, it's hard to break out. But when you see someone who has gotten out of the cycle, you notice. As you move toward greater health, get ready for people to ask you what you've been doing. You will explain, and some people will understand; others won't. Stick with it. Over time, more and more people will say, "I like what you're doing. I want to try it."

My hope is that this book has led you to those same words. As you have read how our wellness program launched and progressed, I hope you are encouraged to implement some of the strategies shared in this book in your own company. My hope is that my own story and the stories of our employees have encouraged you to continue to form your own health story, one that others will want to mirror. After all, it starts with YOU.

A FINAL CALL TO ACTION

Finally, I want to encourage you to be the change you want to see and to remember that you can accomplish anything you set your mind to doing. Stay in the moment, and don't forget to have fun!

I would love to hear about your progress. We are all in this journey together, so let me know how I can help you.

Connect with me on LinkedIn.

—Joshua DeTillio

ABOUT THE AUTHOR

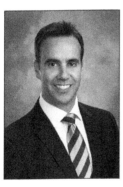 JOSHUA DETILLIO is chief administrative officer at Gulf Coast Medical Center and an adjunct professor at Florida Gulf Coast University. He attended the US Military Academy, served for five years in the Army, received master's degrees in business administration and public health from Vanderbilt and Harvard, and is certified in plant-based nutrition through Cornell. Josh is also a Fellow with the American College of Healthcare Executives.

Passionate about healthy living, Josh was a swimmer at West Point, has competed in more than fifty triathlons, meditates, surfs, is learning tai chi, and does Crossfit and yoga. He lives in Florida with his wife and two children.

Made in the USA
Las Vegas, NV
25 March 2023

69664633R00085